Running a Safe
and Successful
Acupuncture Clinic

CW00550333

For Elsevier:

Commissioning Editor: **Karen Morley**
Development Editors: **Louise Allsop, Kerry McGechie**
Project Manager: **Emma Riley**
Design Direction: **Andy Chapman**
Illustrator: **Michael Courtney**

Running a Safe and Successful Acupuncture Clinic

Hong Zhen Zhu

Dr TCM, RAc (Canada) MD (China)

Traditional Chinese Medicine Practitioner and Clinical Instructor, Victoria, BC, Canada

Foreword by
William R Morris
OMD MSEd LAc
President, American Association of Oriental Medicine

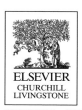

ELSEVIER
CHURCHILL
LIVINGSTONE

EDINBURGH   LONDON   NEW YORK   OXFORD   PHILADELPHIA   ST LOUIS   SYDNEY   TORONTO   2006

ELSEVIER
CHURCHILL
LIVINGSTONE

An imprint of Elsevier Limited

© 2006, Elsevier Ltd. All rights reserved.

First published 2006

ISBN 0 443 10088 8

British Library Cataloguing in Publication Data
A catalogue record for this book is available from the British Library

Library of Congress Cataloging in Publication Data
A catalogue record for this book is available from the Library of Congress

---

NOTICE

Knowledge and best practice in this field are constantly changing. As new research and experience broaden our knowledge, changes in practice, treatment and drug therapy may become necessary or appropriate. Readers are advised to check the most current information provided (i) on procedures featured or (ii) by the manufacturer of each product to be administered, to verify the recommended dose or formula, the method and duration of administration, and contraindications. It is the responsibility of the practitioners, relying on their own experience and knowledge of the patient, to make diagnoses, to determine dosages and the best treatment for each individual patient, and to take all appropriate safety precautions.
To the fullest extent of the law, neither the publisher nor the author assumes any liability for any injury and/or damage.

The Publisher

Printed in China

Contents

Section One: Safety and risk management

Section Two: Ethics and interpersonal skills

Section Three: Professional development and clinic management

Running a Safe and Successful Acupuncture Clinic

"Running a Safe and Successful Acupuncture Clinic represents a distinct step forward for the practice of acupuncture as a clinical discipline . . . Zhu's original contribution will enhance the professional practice of acupuncture and Oriental medicine".
William R Morris, OMD, MSEd, LAc
President, American Association of Oriental Medicine

"It is amazing that Dr Hong Zhen Zhu has taken the trouble to review acupuncture mishaps in such detail and to advise about the ways to avoid them. This is a remarkable book. Dr Zhu has created a masterpiece that should become the standard text for all students and practitioners of acupuncture and TCM. From potential complications, and techniques to avoid them, to the nuances of relating to patients and the ethics of practice, he has left no stone unturned."
Linda M Rapson, MD, CAFCI, Chair, Complementary Medicine Section, Ontario Medical Association, Canada. President, Ontario Society of Physicians for Complementary Medicine,
Executive President, Acupuncture Foundation of Canada Institute and Medical Director, Rapson Pain and Acupuncture Clinic.

"What a wonderful book! The text is what has been missing in acupuncture/TCM education for the student and neophyte practitioner – and is also a good read for the experienced practitioner to refresh and reflect. The book is testament to Dr Zhu's rich experience in the dual role of practitioner and educator. He understands and delivers the information that, until this book, has not been readily available and easily readable and referenced by students and new practitioners. This book is very much needed in today's educational system – and the sooner it gets out there the better!"
Mary Watterson, Dr TCM, Reg Ac Member of Standards of Education and Examination Committees, College of TCM Practitioners and Acupuncturists of BC, Canada. Founding Member, North American Council for Acupuncture and Oriental Medicine.

"This book is very engaging and holds your interest. That is because it is not too technical and it is fun to read. Situations one commonly encounters in clinical practice are presented comprehensively in simple and clear language so before you know it you have read the whole book . . . It serves as a great handbook for re-examining my practice. This book is the amalgamation of the author's rich clinical experience in the West and his business savvy. It is a long awaited text indispensable for all practitioners."
Junji Mizutani, Chief Editor and Director of NAJOM (the North American Journal of Oriental Medicine).

"The issue of safety will always be one of the highest priorities in the field of acupuncture and Oriental medicine. Dr. Zhu's book on safety, patient/practitioner issues, and basic information regarding one's practice offers superb information on a variety of topics that affect every practitioner. His case studies are practical and most informative. This book should be in all college libraries and practitioners' offices."
Elizabeth A Goldblatt, PhD, MPA/HA, Provost/VPAA at the American College of Traditional Chinese Medicine (ACTCM), former President of the Council of College of Acupuncture and Oriental Medicine, USA, and the Oregon College of Oriental Medicine, Portland, USA.

About the author

Hong Zhen Zhu, Dr TCM, RAc (Canada), MD (China) is a master of the art of traditional Chinese medicine and a treasury of expertise and compassion, based on 30 years of practice and teaching in China and Canada. He earned his medical degree at Chongqing University of Medical Science, China, where he studied under professors and doctors who pioneered the fusion between traditional Chinese and Western medicine, which guides his practice to this day.

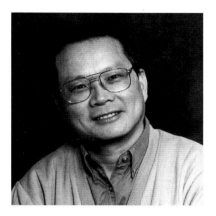

Dr Zhu's experience ranges from training barefoot doctors in the Three Gorges region of the Yangtze River during the Cultural Revolution, to working as a general physician practising both Western and Eastern medicine at the famous Ren Ji Hospital in Chongqing, established more than a century ago by Canadian missionaries.

Dr Zhu, who now has a thriving Traditional Chinese Medicine (TCM) practice in Victoria, BC, Canada, has published numerous articles and research papers in medical magazines, journals and newspapers in China, Canada and the United States. He has also been an instructor, clinical supervisor and president of the Canadian College of Acupuncture and Oriental Medicine.

Throughout this book, you will feel his generous spirit and his profound knowledge.

Dr Zhu is also the author of *Building a Jade Screen: Better Health with Chinese Medicine* (Penguin Canada).

Contributors

SUSAN BROWN, DTCM, LicAc (UK) is now retired from private practice in Victoria, BC, Canada, where she also taught at the Canadian College of Acupuncture and Oriental Medicine.

HEATHER BURY, Dr TCM, has a private acupuncture and TCM practice in Comox, BC, Canada, and teaches anatomy and Oriental medical theory at Windsong School of Healing in Campbell River, BC, Canada. She also spends two months each winter teaching at the Rebalancing Bodywork residential school in Costa Rica.

XIA CHENG, MD (China), PhD, RAc, earned a PhD in Medicine, specialising in acupuncture and chronomedicine (Chengdu University of TCM) and has been a physician, herbalist, acupuncturist and researcher for more than 20 years. She has taught at colleges in Europe, Canada and China, published several TCM works, and continues to be involved in the process of regulating acupuncture and TCM in the province of Alberta, Canada. She is the founder and president of the Canadian Institute of Traditional Chinese Medicine and the director of the BodyMind Synergy Health Centre, both in Calgary, Canada.

LOUISE DEMOREST, Dr TCM, is an acupuncturist and herbalist with a private practice in Richmond, BC, Canada. Her advanced studies in China and Japan included acupuncture, Japanese massage, Zen Shiatsu and herbology. She is certified in the acu-detox protocols of the National Acupuncture Detoxification Association, and has been involved in research on drug addiction and multiple sclerosis. Dr Demorest is a former president of the Acupuncture Association of British Columbia and sits on the North American Council on Acupuncture and Oriental Medicine.

DAVID IP, RAc, DTCM, DAc, trained in TCM theory and practice in Calgary, Canada. He interned at the Zhejiang College of Traditional Chinese Medicine, the largest TCM school in the world, in the city of Hangzhou, China, home of the famous and scenic West Lake. David Ip now has his own West Lake Clinic in Regina, Canada, where his treatment specialties include chronic pain relief and adjunct therapy for patients receiving conventional medical treatment.

CHRISTOPHER LAM, MD, is a Western-trained medical doctor and physician acupuncturist with an integrated general practice in Victoria, BC, Canada. He is also past president, Association of Complementary Physicians of British Columbia, and a Clinical Instructor in the Department of Family Practice, Faculty of Medicine, University of British Columbia, Vancouver, BC, Canada.

XIAOSHU ZHU, BMed (Nanjing, China) MMed (Nanjing, China), PhD candidate (Sydney, Australia), is a lecturer and clinical coordinator for the Chinese Medicine Program, School of Exercise and Health

Sciences, and a Researcher, Center for Complementary Medicine Research at the University of Western Sydney, Australia. She is also a qualified and registered Chinese Medicine Practitioner, and over the past 20 years has amassed intensive teaching and clinical experience both in China and Australia.

Foreword

The western practice of acupuncture has progressed beyond its early roots when Harviell introduced *The Secrets of Chinese Medicine, Consisting of the Perfect Knowledge* to Europe in 1671 and Benjamin Franklin's great grandson Dr Franklin Bache wrote the first US medical acupuncture article, entitled *Memoirs on Acupuncture* in 1825. Given these initial forays into the arcane methods of the east, acupuncture literature remained rare until James Reston, a reporter for *The Times*, witnessed a surgery using acupuncture anesthesia while traveling with President Nixon. This sparked interest in acupuncture and English language translations from the great body of Chinese literature. Then, subsequent to the increasing popularity, research and growth of accredited degree programs in acupuncture, the FDA reclassified the acupuncture needles from experimental devices to Class II medical devices in 1996. In a similar vein, *Running a Safe and Successful Acupuncture Clinic* represents a distinct step forward for the practice of acupuncture as a clinical discipline.

Hong Zhen Zhu is to be lauded for bringing an essential discussion of risk and ethics in the practice of acupuncture to the foreground. With case histories and evidence he discusses an array of adverse events along with useful management strategies and referral criteria. There are clear descriptions of anatomical structure and the symptoms that can occur after inadvertent puncture of vulnerable structures such as the organs or nerves. The cases discuss the very real risks of inappropriate needling methods along with graphic examples of the needling method that caused the complication. Consideration is given to the anatomy and anatomical changes that occur in various disease states that can increase the risk of damage to organs. Although serious complications are rare, the authors share cases that highlight the very real problems that can occur when acupuncture is performed improperly or by under trained personnel.

This is a clearly referenced and evidence based approach to the management and prevention of adverse reactions that can occur in the administration of acupuncture. The discussion includes needling risks based on normal anatomy as well as the risks that are of concern for certain body types and diseases conditions.

The development of ethical concerns has been correlated with the emergence of medical professions within most cultures. While the concern for ethics in medicine has been present since the earliest records in the Persian Hammurabi texts circa 2300 BCE and developed further in the Hippocratic

Oath as well as the writings of the famous Sung Dynasty physician Sun Simiao, the translation of medical ethical discussion from an eastern culture to the west has not received much attention. The author discusses the historic development of ethics through the three treasures of Confucianism, Taoism and Buddhism. He connects it to the practice of acupuncture in the modern clinical settings of the west. It is reasonable to predict that essential materials like this will provide a basis for the development of public policy and protection in the future, especially as it concerns the need for professional level training in acupuncture.

This text will have an impact on the development of standards of practice for acupuncture in the west. The clear discussion of risk involved with the procedures will assist legislators to understand the need for training to a full level of competency. It will assist those practitioners who are forging laws in parts of the world where there are none to establish for the public that the necessary critical dialogues are occurring within the profession such that autonomy is granted and the rights to exercise professional judgment are preserved.

Zhu's original contribution will enhance the professional practice of acupuncture and Oriental Medicine.

William R Morris

Preface

This book will form a valuable addition to the reference library of anyone associated with acupuncture and traditional Chinese medicine (TCM). It is among the first in the English language to amalgamate into one comprehensive work the issues of ethical considerations and risk management, as well as offering in-depth, practical answers to the questions of newly graduated practitioners facing a new set of daunting tasks following their formal education.

Others who will benefit from this book include students, especially in their internship years, looking ahead to starting their own practice. It will make students aware of the serious nature of ethical practice and accident prevention from the very beginning. It takes far more than a knowledge of point location and needling technique to make a good acupuncturist; our responsibility to patients requires taking care at every step. If we cannot always help, at least we will know enough to do no harm.

This book is also helpful for the practitioners who want to deepen their knowledge, whether that is in learning more effective and less painful needle techniques, better clinical management or going to China to study. It goes into great detail in areas of technique because the quality of our practice and the success of our treatments rest on our attention to these small but crucial matters.

Applicants for certification and licensing exams will find the sections on safe and effective needling, infection control and accident prevention in acupuncture and other TCM techniques a useful reference. The book is a new and valuable resource for registration bodies setting licensing and competency standards, as well as for anyone researching legal issues related to the safe and ethical practice of acupuncture.

Emergency and trauma departments of hospitals will want to have this reference on hand for review by their physicians and surgeons, to enhance their knowledge of what injuries can fairly and accurately be attributed to an acupuncture treatment, and when they are only coincident and not related to acupuncture. This will avoid a significant number of misunderstandings that currently arise between Western and TCM practice.

In addition, medical doctors and other health professionals who are incorporating traditional Chinese medicine into their practice will find information to help them connect their knowledge of human physiology with the theory and practice of acupuncture.

2005, Victoria, BC, Canada   *Hong Zhen Zhu*

Acknowledgements

My wife Xiao Feng Li and daughter Judy Zhu have been a constant, daily and faithful support in body and spirit. In addition to their unwavering encouragement, they have also uncomplainingly dealt with many mundane tasks such as research, typing, proof reading, computer problems and the regular and crucial contribution of nourishing and comforting meals!

The creation of a book of this scope has required skills that go far beyond technical writing ability. As editor, Sherry Lepage has been one part writer, one part psychologist and one part mind reader. Sherry is a writer and filmmaker who specializes in health education projects, several of which have won awards in international competition, as well as social issue and cultural documentaries which have been broadcast across Canada. Over the year that we have worked together on this book, we have enjoyed many fruitful discussions about complementary medicine philosophies and the interplay of cultures. Her questions have sometimes sent me scurrying home to do more research and expand my own thinking. Sherry's entire family has lent its support, especially her daughter, Sara Cowan, whose advice on what psychology students like and dislike about university textbooks helped us with many details. The fact that this is the second book we have happily collaborated on says a great deal about how much I value our partnership. I feel very fortunate to be able to call on her skills and her friendship.

The assistance of Heather Bury, Dr TCM, has been invaluable, especially in the formative stages of the book. As a skilled practitioner, as well as a former student of mine, she contributed many excellent ideas about content and structure, and edited much of the original manuscript. As the book has grown and developed, Heather's international teaching experience has widened its scope, and she has been extremely generous with her knowledge and advice. Her many contributions are woven throughout the text, but are especially evident in the sections on following up with herbal prescriptions, the schools, styles and cultural context of Chinese medicine in the West and marketing and publicity.

I am also profoundly grateful for the assistance of Louise Demorest, Dr TCM, whose background as a leader of professional bodies in the field of acupuncture has given her a comprehensive understanding of ethics and professional practices, which she has contributed to this book. She raised a number of important issues, from legal questions to technique, which kept us busy making sure these important matters were properly covered. As an experienced practitioner, she has also offered so many suggestions that if we were to take them all we would still be writing! As a member of the North American Council on Acupuncture and Oriental Medicine, Louise has many international connections in the field, which she has been kind enough to share, giving the book a wider usefulness.

Christopher Lam, MD and physician acupuncturist, embodies in spirit and practice the reason why the integration of Chinese and Western medicine can be greater than the sum of its parts! His contribution in Section 2 should be required reading for every medical practitioner, Western and Eastern. I also greatly appreciate his help in locating some of the anatomical illustration references and correcting proofs.

This project has benefited greatly from the assistance of Xia Cheng MD (China), PhD, RAc, who brings her vast knowledge, many academic qualifications and international experience as a practitioner and educator. I thank her for her contributions, which include a historical perspective of the development of ethics in TCM, as well as suggestions on clinical management, style and customs of treatment, the use of herbs, and study in China. I also appreciate her generosity of spirit in introducing me to her colleague David Ip.

I would also like to express my appreciation to David Ip, RAc, DTCM, DAc, for his excellent and well thought-out contributions to the ethics section, particularly the articles on dealing with patients who face difficult health issues, and on professional ethics.

My deep thanks to Mary Watterson, Dr TCM, who as a leader and pioneer in the registration of acupuncture and development of standards of practice in Canada has been extremely helpful in providing communication and networking information. She has responded to every request with grace.

I am very grateful to Linda Rapson, MD, chair of the Complementary Medicine Section of the Ontario Medical Association and president of the Ontario Society of Physicians for Complementary Medicine, for volunteering to undertake a detailed technical review of the manuscript, and in the process, correcting a number of awkward translations of Western medical terms.

Across the Pacific Ocean, I extend my thanks to Xiaoshu Zhu, Dr TCM, RAc and an educator at the University of Western Sydney. Despite her extensive travels between Australia and China, she somehow managed to squeeze in the time to update the section on study in China.

And thanks also to Susan Brown, DTCM, LicAc (UK), for allowing me to use her article on sexual ethics.

Finally, for their assistance in many ways, from lending research materials and sharing information about issues in their practice, to modelling for illustrations to taking photographs, I thank the following people for their kindness and generosity: Winston Wei, Phyllis Wei, Maureen Renier Dr TCM, Tamara Kitzmann RAc, Tingting Jiang Dr TCM, Bonnie E. Robinson Dr TCM, Stephanie Curran RAc, TCMP, Charlene West RAc, Alexandra Zowisza RAc, Nancy Issenman Dr TCM, James Thom, Wang Zhuxing MD (China), Hong Tao MD (China), Wang Xie, Lincoln Jiang, Wei Zhu, June Beckford MA Dr TCM, Susan Rundans BA and Sylvia Weinstock.

SECTION 1

Safety and risk management

Section Contents

INTRODUCTION

Despite the growing popularity of traditional Chinese medicine (TCM) in non-Asian countries, there is still a great deal of misunderstanding in Western conventional medicine about the way acupuncture actually works, and which techniques are considered to be standard practice when applied by properly trained, competent acupuncturists. Also, members of the public generally lack enough knowledge of TCM to know whether the practitioners they are seeing are, in fact, trained and competent. These factors give rise to a couple of misapprehensions in the way acupuncture is sometimes perceived in the West: either as a kind of folk medicine that is essentially harmless, or, at the opposite extreme, a discipline that is only safe when practised by those with a medical degree.

The fact that in many jurisdictions the practice of acupuncture is entirely unregulated means that there are more accidents than there should be, even though serious adverse effects are quite rare, especially when compared with scores of thousands of deaths annually from conventional drug therapy. Whereas adverse drug reactions account for 3–7% of hospitalizations and 0.5–0.9% of deaths, the incidence of adverse effects from acupuncture is very small, considering the millions of patients treated each year.

Let us first distinguish an error from an accident. An error could be a stuck needle, a bent needle, a small bruise or bleeding, or the patient feeling weak and nauseated after a treatment. Every acupuncturist – especially in the early years of practice – will inadvertently cause these problems on occasion. Sometimes a medication the patient is taking will have an unexpected effect when combined with acupuncture. These conditions are not considered to be accidents as they are simple to handle and do not have long-term consequences for the patient.

Acupuncture-related accidents are more serious than errors, because they:

- create long-term consequences for a patient (for example, leading to a series of operations)
- worsen a patient's original condition (for example, if an emphysema patient with a pneumothorax developed scar tissue that considerably aggravated a lung problem)
- disable a patient, or
- cause death.

The main causes of acupuncture accidents are: incorrect depth/angle of needle insertion, insufficient anatomical knowledge, failure to follow antiseptic procedures at any stage of the process, failure to focus the mind on the treatment or to observe the patient carefully, and treating a patient who is too weak or one who has a condition that contraindicates acupuncture (a haemophiliac, for example).

Internationally, the acupuncture field pays a considerable amount of attention to accident prevention and publishes cases in journals. In China, from

1949 to 1994, there were 878 significant or serious accidents reported, 23 of them fatal. One of these deaths involved a severe allergic reaction caused by medication injected through an acupoint; the remaining 22 were traumatic injuries. Brain, spinal cord and central nervous system damage accounted for 10 of these. There were four fatal heart injuries, two cases of haemorrhage from arterial punctures and one death caused by an injury to the trachea. Severe pneumothorax killed five patients (Zhou Jianwei 1995). Of course we have no way of knowing how many incidents occurred that were not reported or made public.

In 2001, researchers in the United Kingdom reported their conclusion that acupuncture is a relatively safe treatment. Their opinion was based on a mail-in survey of treatment data collected from 574 professional acupuncturists: about 30% of the total membership of the British Acupuncture Council. The survey covered 4 weeks and 34 407 treatments. In that time, no serious adverse events – those requiring admission to hospital, prolonging a hospital stay, or causing permanent disability or death – were reported.

There were 43 significant minor adverse events, such as severe nausea, fainting, an unacceptable level of local pain and bruising and psychological reactions. This amounts to a rate of 1.3 per 1000 treatments. Of these, three accidents could have been avoided: needles were left in two patients and a third received moxa burns.

Minor local reactions such as mild bruising, pain or slight bleeding were reported in just over 3% of the treatments. In 15% of the cases, patients experienced mild transient reactions, most commonly feeling relaxed or feeling energized after treatment (MacPherson et al 2001).

Although some papers define 'adverse' as any unintended or non-therapeutic effect, in many cases, such as a patient with insomnia, anxiety or high stress levels, relaxation would be one of the treatment objectives, so in our discussion here we do not consider this a negative event. However, relaxation – in other words, prolonged de qi – could be dangerous if the patient is driving immediately after treatment.

In another British survey, 78 acupuncturists – all doctors or physiotherapists – reported events in 6.8% of the 31 822 treatments given during the reporting period. Forty-three significant minor events – bleeding, needling pain and aggravation of symptoms – occurred; only a third of these interfered with patients' daily activities. Again, there were no serious adverse events (White et al 2001). A small survey of practitioners in Germany in the early 1980s yielded similar results.

American medical acupuncturist James K. Rotchford MD concludes that serious complications of acupuncture, such as cardiac tamponade, hepatitis and pneumothorax, are quite rare, occurring in about 1 in 5000 cases. He bases this opinion on his own experience of approximately 30 000 treatments, as well as literature reviews such as that of Palle Rosted (1996). Rotchford believes practitioners must be aware of how to prevent and recognize these events, but they are so unusual that it is not necessary to discuss them in detail with patients.

Detailed anatomical knowledge and proper training of practitioners is essential in avoiding serious complications associated with acupuncture. A study in Australia found that the incidence of adverse events was 2.07 per year among practitioners with less than 1 year of training. The accident rate dropped to .92 adverse events per year in the group of practitioners who had received 49 to 60 months of training (Bensoussan & Myers 1996).

Public safety is best served where solid standards of competent practice are set by a regulatory body such as a College of Acupuncture, which ensures continuing education of practitioners and has the power to withdraw the licence of any acupuncturist found to be incompetent.

Even a casual review of the literature leads us to the conclusion that most accidents occur at the hands of practitioners who are not sufficiently trained in how to prevent adverse events, to recognize them if they occur, or to take appropriate action if a patient is injured. The following sections will address these issues.

NOTES ON MEASUREMENTS AND MERIDIANS

Measurements given for needle lengths, depths of insertion and distances for locating points in acupuncture are often puzzling; different forms are used in various texts. Some references use 'cun'; at other times inches or centimetres are used.

FIXED CUN

To clarify, there is in fact more than one kind of cun. One is a unit of length that, converted into Western measurements, is 33.333 mm or 1.3123 inches. When used in reference to acupuncture needles, a 1 cun needle is in fact 25 mm in length, a ½ cun needle is 13 mm long, a 2 cun needle is 50 mm and a 3 cun one is 75 mm because of the limitations of manufacturing technology. These measurements refer only to the shaft and do not include the handle.

AVERAGE CUN

In this book, when referring to the depth of insertion, for the sake of consistency the length of the needle is used to indicate the measurement. This is still an imperfect solution, however, as there may be variations in correct depth depending on the amount of fat and muscle on a particular person at a particular point, or whether the patient is a child, a burly adult or a frail elderly person. Like the so-called 'standard' dose of a medication, insertion depths given in this book are an average, which practitioners may have to adjust on the basis of their best judgement.

INDIVIDUAL CUN

When locating a point, we also use the unit of cun, but this is different from the needle cun. The point location measurement is called a 'tong shen cun', which means a certain part of the patient's body is divided into sections of equal length, each of which is taken as one proportional or identical unit for measurement. This of course means that a cun on one person is not the same measurement as it is on another person of different build.

In this book, when we talk about the needle we have no hesitation in specifying the cun as the exact measurement, but when we are discussing point location we mean tong shen cun. This is why point location distances are not converted to Western scientific measurements.

Various references use different names for some points. To avoid confusion here is a list of point and meridian names chosen for this book:

- Lung – LU
- Large Intestine – LI
- Stomach – ST
- Spleen – SP
- Heart – HT
- Small Intestine – SI
- Bladder – BL
- Kidney – KI
- Pericardium – PC
- Triple Burner (also known as Triple Warmer, Triple Energizer or San Jiao) – TB
- Liver – LIV
- Gall Bladder – GB
- Governor Vessel – Du
- Conception Vessel – Ren
- Extra points – Ex.

References

Bensoussan A, Myers SP. Towards a safer choice: the practice of traditional Chinese medicine in Australia. Sydney Australia Macarthur 1996

MacPherson H, Thomas K, Walters S et al. A prospective survey of adverse events and treatment reactions following 34 000 consultations with professional acupuncturists. *Acupuncture in Medicine* 2001, 19(2):93-102

Rosted P. Literature survey of reported adverse effects associated with acupuncture treatment. *American Journal of Acupuncture* 1996, 24:27-34

White A, Hayhoe S, Hart A, Ernst E et al. Survey of adverse events following acupuncture: a prospective study of 32,000 Consultations. *Acupuncture in Medicine* 2001, 19(2) 84–92

Zhou Jianwei. Acupuncture Injuries and Safe Needling Techniques for Dangerous Points. Sichuan Science and Technology Publishing House 1995 Chengdu

Nervous system and blood vessels

1

SUBARACHNOID HAEMORRHAGE

Of 200 cases of subarachnoid haemorrhage reported in a literature review, 10 were the result of acupuncture accidents. The rest were caused by aneurysms, strokes, high blood pressure, arteriosclerosis or trauma. The significant number of reported incidents warrants careful attention to technique to prevent this serious, and potentially fatal, outcome.

Case study 1.1

A male, aged 57, sought acupuncture treatment to relieve spasms in his right-side facial muscles. On the first treatment, points in the neck and occipital region were used with no problems. Two days later, the patient returned for his second treatment, and the same group of points was employed. Once the needles had been inserted, he felt an electric shock sensation down the right side of his body, from head to foot. Nevertheless, the needles were left in place for 5 minutes before they were removed. The patient then reported dizziness and nausea, and after an hour developed a severe headache and vomited twice. He was taken to hospital, where his blood pressure was found to be 190/110 mmHg. The physician diagnosed hypertension, and a further examination was scheduled for the headache. The afternoon of the same day, back at home, the patient once again vomited twice. The following day, the headache was worse, and the man's neck was stiff and immobile. When there was no improvement after 3 more days, he was admitted to hospital. Tests revealed blood in the cerebral fluid, and a meningeal irritation test was positive. Diagnosis was that acupuncture accident had caused a subarachnoid haemorrhage. After 3 weeks of treatment the man recovered completely (Chen et al 1985).

Case study 1.2

An unusual case report comes from Japan, where a 33-year-old woman suddenly developed severe occipital headaches. X-rays revealed a fine gold needle, about 1.5 cm. long, between the C1 and C2 vertebrae. It had been in the woman's body since an acupuncture treatment 30 years earlier, and had eventually pierced the spinal nerve root through the dural vein, causing subarachnoid haemorrhage. The needle was removed, and after surgery the pain the woman had experienced while moving her neck disappeared (Murata et al 1990).

Related acupoints

Du-5 to Du-16, especially Du-15 and Du-16
GB-20
Ex. Hua Tuo Jia Ji, Ex. An Mian, Ex. Yi Ming

Discussion of subarachnoid haemorrhage

The subarachnoid is a space surrounding the entire central nerve system (Fig. 1.1). It is located between the arachnoid membrane and the deepest meninx – the pia mater layer. Many small blood vessels are attached to the surface of the pia mater, and these vessels nourish the underlying cells of the brain and spinal cord. The subarachnoid space is maintained by delicate, web-like strands that connect the arachnoid membrane and pia mater. This web-like membrane spreads over the surface of the central nervous system and follows the irregular contours of the brain and spinal cord. The subarachnoid space holds a quantity of cerebrospinal fluid. If an acupuncture needle pierces any of the small vessels on the pia mater, blood will leak into the subarachnoid space.

In addition, it is possible to puncture one of two major vessels: the vertebral artery, which enters the cranium through the great occipital foramen, and one of its main branches, the anterior spinal artery, which goes into the skull via the medullary bulb.

The acupuncture literature contains many reports of haemorrhage at the base of the brain caused by incorrect needling of Du-15, Du-16, GB-20, Ex. Yi

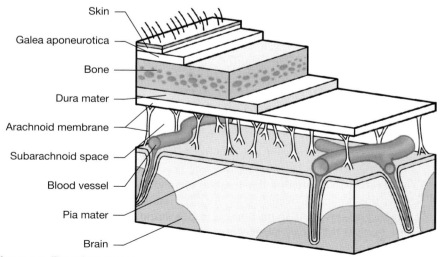

Skin
Galea aponeurotica
Bone
Dura mater
Arachnoid membrane
Subarachnoid space
Blood vessel
Pia mater
Brain

Figure 1.1 The subarachnoid space.

Ming or Ex. An Mian. Also, because the arachnoid membrane covers the spinal cord as well as the brain itself, by puncturing points along the spine we can also cause a subarachnoid haemorrhage. For example, there are cases in which this accident resulted from needling Du-13. The symptoms and progress of such an injury are the same as those of a spinal cord injury: blood will leak into the cerebrospinal fluid and eventually fill the cavity, irritating the meningeal membrane. Without proper and immediate treatment, this can cause death.

What to do in case of subarachnoid haemorrhage

Suspect a puncture if, when treating the points listed above, a patient complains of sudden sharp pain around the needle site, an electric shock sensation, or develops a sudden severe headache in the occipital area, nausea, vomiting, confusion or sleepiness.

If the injury is minor, the confusion and sleepiness will pass off shortly. If symptoms continue, or the patient loses consciousness, this is a clear sign that there is bleeding into the subarachnoid cavity.

Stop the treatment immediately and remove all needles if any of these symptoms arise. Do not allow the patient to sit or stand if you suspect a haemorrhage; call for an ambulance right away. Patients with subarachnoid haemorrhage need to be in hospital. Diagnosis will be made with a computerised tomography (CT) scan, and lumbar puncture to look for blood in the cerebrospinal fluid. Prompt medical treatment usually results in a full recovery, as long as the punctured vessel is a small one. A puncture of the major vertebral artery (which has happened through GB-20) may be fatal.

Prevention of subarachnoid haemorrhage

When we do work on Du-15 and Du-16, special care must be taken with the direction of the needle (Fig. 1.2). Have the patient lie on the stomach or side, and have the chin slightly dropped toward the chest, to relax the neck muscles and expose the treatment area. The tip of the needle should be inserted at a slightly downward angle, pointing toward the mouth. There is more subcutaneous tissue at that spot to protect the sensitive area of the brain, and the angle will prevent the needle from falling into the trap of the foramen magnum. It is more likely the needle will hit this foramen if it is angled more toward the nose.

Conversely, we do want to angle the needle upward toward the tip of the nose when treating GB-20. This way, the needle will be stopped by the skull bone rather than entering the occipital foramen. Some textbooks suggest the practitioner aim the needle tip in the direction of the opposite eyeball when working on this point. In my opinion, it is safest to use the nose as the guideline, because the line of the needle will be more parallel to the side of the head. This ensures the needle will not slip under the edge of the skull. An alternative technique suggested in some texts for treating GB-20 is to insert two needles,

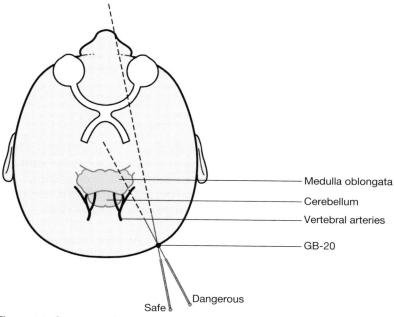

Medulla oblongata

Cerebellum

Vertebral arteries

GB-20

Safe

Dangerous

Figure 1.2 Correct and incorrect needling angle for GB-20. Angling the needle toward the tip of the patient's nose, instead of toward the opposite eyeball, will ensure it does not touch the medulla oblongata.

with the needle tips pointing toward each other. In this way, the needles will remain safely in subcutaneous tissue and muscle.

Practitioners also need to be careful of the depth of insertion on these points. In general, here acupuncturists rarely needle beyond 1 cun, and even less when treating a thin person. A depth of 1.5 cun increases the risk of injury for most people; in a thin person the needle will already be touching the dura mater at this depth. When treating a heavy person, 1.5 cun should be the absolute maximum needle depth.

When needling points at the base of the skull, practitioners must also carefully feel the needle sensation. The needle passes through the skin, subcutaneous tissue, then the nuchal ligament, which is encountered as a resistance. This is the place to stop. If the needle is forced more deeply, it will hit the occipital bone or vertebral body, where it may slip around the edge of the bony structure and into the dura mater. If you feel the needle tip touch bone, back it off slightly.

When treating points over the arachnoid cavity of the spinal cord, the situation is similar. Under the subcutaneous layer there is connective tissue, especially the yellow ligament, which is a tough, leathery layer that resists the needle. Again, this is the place to stop. If the needle seems to be falling into emptiness, it is in the epidural space, and should be pulled back to avoid puncturing the dura mater.

In addition to the needle's angle, depth and sensation, a safe treatment in such sensitive areas requires the patient's cooperation and readiness to accept the needles. Some injuries have occurred when patients such as children, or people with mental problems, have been held down while needles were inserted, then moved abruptly. There are always safer alternative points and techniques that practitioners can choose in such cases.

SPINAL CORD INJURY

Injuries to the spinal cord from acupuncture are unusual but serious. According to Peuker & Gronemeyer (2001), these rank with pneumothorax as the most frequently reported serious complications of acupuncture. In terms of their actual incidence, in Rampes & James' (1995) summary of 395 instances of acupuncture-related complications, only a handful involved injury to the spinal cord.

In this section we examine transient injuries resulting from spinal concussion or obstruction and, more seriously, spinal contusion.

Case study 1.3

A 30-year-old woman who had been suffering from schizophrenia for 7 years was admitted to a hospital in China on 3 January 1970. In addition to medication and other treatments, she was given acupuncture. She had her seventh acupuncture session a month after her admission, on 3 February. A needle was inserted into Du-14, with electrical stimulation. After 4 minutes of gentle stimulation, an intermittent pulse was administered. The patient's limbs suddenly became paralysed and flaccid, and her face was pale with a purplish tinge. Treatment was stopped and cardiopulmonary resuscitation (CPR) was performed for an hour, but the patient died. An autopsy found an acupuncture hole in the spine near the junction between the cervical and thoracic segments.

In analysing this famous case, it is clear that two factors combined to cause the patient's death. First, the needle at Du-14 was placed at a depth and angle that allowed it to puncture the spinal cord. Secondly, the strong electrical pulse feeding directly into the spinal cord was transmitted into the brain stem, causing cardiac and respiratory arrest (Liu 1981).

Case study 1.4

Another case, which ended more happily for the patient, involved a 43-year-old man who had been receiving ongoing treatment for lower back pain. There were no adverse effects until his 12th treatment, during which he lost consciousness and became paralysed below midthoracic level. A magnetic resonance imaging (MRI) scan showed a 15 cm long lesion in the midthoracic section of the spinal cord. The patient had a full recovery after medical treatment (Ilham et al 1995).

Related acupoints

Du-5 to Du-16, especially Du-13–Du-16
Ex. Hua Tuo Jia Ji

Discussion of spinal cord injury

The spinal cord is a long and fragile part of the nervous system that functions as a communications link between the brain and the rest of the body. It begins at the bottom of the brain stem and, cradled by the vertebrae that make up the spinal column, runs down the centre of the back to the level of the first lumbar vertebra, almost to the bottom of the spine. There are 31 pairs of nerves that branch off from the cord and out through the grooves, or foramina, between the vertebrae.

The cord itself has a central core of grey matter, surrounded by white matter through which nerve tracts run. The ascending tracts, or sensory nerves, carry sensory information from the body's peripheral receptors to the brain; descending tracts take motor impulses from the brain to the muscles and glands. The spinal cord also contains nerve pathways that are involved in involuntary movement of muscles that control the heart rate, respiration and digestion, among other functions.

Like the brain, the spinal cord is wrapped by three layers of tissue known collectively as meninges – the pia mater, the arachnoid mater and the tough, leathery dura mater – and cushioned by cerebrospinal fluid.

The main cause of spinal cord injury from acupuncture is incorrect depth and angle of needle placement. The distance from the surface of the skin to the spinal cord ranges from 30 to 50 mm. Some medical researchers write that it is as little as 25–45 mm. The distance depends on the patient's body type. The points Du-5 to Du-16, going up from the first lumbar vertebra, are all located just below each spinous process, in the tiny gap between the vertebrae. If the tip of the needle is aimed at an oblique upward angle, it will slide into these intervertebral foramina, and puncture the spinal cord.

In the literature, the points most often associated with spinal cord injury are Du-13, Du-14 and Du-15, especially Du-14, which is located between the vertebrae C7 and T1. The spinal cord segment of T1–T2 lies directly under the acupoint Du-14. If a puncture occurs here, the injury will affect sensory and motor functions controlled by this part of the spinal cord.

The 17 Ex. Hua Tuo Jia Ji points are located 0.5 cun lateral to the spinal column, at the level of the lower border of each spinous process from T1 to L5. If the direction and depth of the needle are wrong, the tip of the needle can slip sideways into the channel between the vertebrae, and come in contact with the spinal cord.

Of the 10 cases of spinal cord injury collected by Peuker & Gronemeyer (2001), six were caused by direct injury. (The others resulted from migration of needle fragments.)

In the early 1970s, as China began to open up to the West, its government wanted to use the amazing technique of acupuncture as a way to impress foreign visitors and governments. Mao's functionaries decided everyone should get on the acupuncture bandwagon – from barefoot doctors to People's Liberation Army soldiers. Their patients were often people with hearing and speech impairments who, if cured, could then praise Chairman Mao's leadership. People with mental illnesses such as schizophrenia were also chosen for treatment.

It is true that acupuncture can be effective in these cases. However, most of these so-called practitioners were not properly trained, and many assumed that the deeper the acupuncture and the stronger the de qi the better the treatment. Many serious injuries resulted from this ignorance. I personally witnessed this as some of the patients who had been damaged by these amateurs came for medical treatment to the Chongqing hospital where I was practising at that time. This political misuse of acupuncture is the reason for the unusually large number of spinal cord injuries and subarachnoid haemorrhages reported in China during the early 1970s.

What to do in case of spinal cord injury

The signs and symptoms of a spinal cord injury are related to the degree of injury. If the needle has merely touched the spinal cord, this spinal concussion – a transient conductive obstruction – would have little effect on the structure of the spinal cord tissue. Symptoms in this case would include sensory disorders in the affected segment: loss of pain or temperature sensation, or the onset of numbness. There might also be segmental motor dysfunction, such as flaccid hemiplegia or paralysis of limbs, faecal or urinary incontinence, or retention of urine, if the sphincter muscles of the rectum or bladder have been affected. Tendon reflexes would disappear temporarily.

General symptoms include dizziness, fatigue, aches all over the body and occasionally a temporary loss of consciousness from shock. All of these would pass off in a few minutes to several hours, although in some cases the patient would be left with a limp for a few days. The symptoms would not recur.

However, such a patient should be checked by a physician to make sure the injury is no more serious than it seems. As long as the needle has not punctured the cord itself, a cerebrospinal fluid exam will be normal. Several days of bed rest should take care of the situation. During this time, the patient should be under the observation of a family member or friend, and should not drive. Any change of consciousness, pulse, respiration, or symptoms that worsen should be reported to a physician or the local emergency department.

A spinal contusion, also known as spinal shock, is a more serious injury. This means one or more needles have punctured the meninges and have gone into the spinal cord itself. Pathological changes to the cord may include oedema, bleeding and malacosis, and necrosis of tissue at the puncture site. Segmental functional disorders resulting from a serious puncture include paralysis, limping and loss of muscle tone. Sensory dysfunction will be more severe and of longer duration than in a milder injury.

In extreme cases, signs of spinal shock are dropping blood pressure, a high fever and rapid pulse. This is an emergency; acupuncture treatment should cease immediately and the patient should be transported to hospital. A cerebrospinal fluid exam will show red blood cells or other abnormal cells, indicating a puncture of the spinal cord. In hospital, if there is internal bleeding or a haematoma, the patient may need surgery to repair the injury. If surgery is not necessary, diuretics, antibiotics and possibly corticosteroids may be prescribed. After recovery from the acute symptoms, the patient may still need physiotherapy, massage, acupuncture or other rehabilitation to regain full sensory and motor functions. Generally, the patient will be back to normal in approximately a month. In extremely rare cases, full recovery has taken as long as 6 months.

Prevention of spinal cord injury

When needling Governor Vessel (Du) points, it is safest to use a perpendicular rather than an oblique angle. This way, the tip of the needle will not be inclined to slide into the channel between the vertebrae and possibly contact the spinal cord; instead, it will be stopped by the spinous process of the bottom vertebra. Contrary to the advice of some other texts, a perpendicular insertion will achieve an effective de qi sensation in people of most body types.

For points such as Ex. Hua Tuo Jia Ji, which are approached from either side of the spine, we try to get the tip of the needle into the spinalis muscle. If the needle's angle is too acute relative to the surface of the back, again there is danger of it sliding into the gap. In this case the desired angle is a minimum of 60° from the skin; if the needle goes too far it will be stopped by a vertebra.

Practitioners also need to pay attention to depth of insertion. For both groups of points just discussed, in people of average body types the depth should be no more than 1 cun, regardless of the size of needle chosen. For patients who are heavier or more muscled, we can place the needle more deeply – between 1 and 1.5 cun. Of course, when treating people who are very small or emaciated, we will go to less than 1 cun.

Pay close attention to needle sensation. When treating Du points, the needle goes through the skin, then subcutaneous tissue, then into supraspinal and interspinal ligaments. Under the Ex. Hua Tuo Jia Ji points, there are lumbodorsal fasciae instead of ligaments. In either case, when you feel the needle hitting the tougher tissue, stop. If you continue to push the needle through these tissues, it will punch through to the epidural space – in other words, into the vertebral canal – which will feel like empty space. Back the needle off immediately, and do not stimulate it.

These groups of points are commonly used in treating poststroke patients. Because of the lack of quick response in people who've had strokes, older text-books advocated strong manual or electrical stimulation to encourage de qi. We now know that a delayed de qi is fine. Wait 3 to 5 minutes, then gently stimu-late the needles. Forcing a response could result in damage to the spinal cord.

In treating patients who've had strokes or accidents, we often use electri-cal stimulation on these two groups of points. It is important to start with a low threshold of stimulation, and raise it in very slow, small increments to allow the patient to adjust to each change. If the electrical pulse is cranked up too quickly, it may cause a muscle spasm that could drive the needle further into the tissue and possibly into the spinal cord.

PERIPHERAL NERVE INJURY

The peripheral nerve system includes spinal and cranial nerves. There are 12 pairs of cranial nerves, all of which originate deep in the grey matter of the brain. These nerves control the sensory and motor functioning of the head, face, neck, trunk and some parts of the inner organs.

There are 31 pairs of spinal nerves, which correspond to the regions of the spine through which they pass: 8 cervical pairs, 12 dorsal, 5 lumbar, 5 sacral and 1 pair of coccygeal nerves. Each spinal nerve comes out of two roots: one anterior (motor) and the other posterior (sensory). The anterior roots form a nerve plexus, which is a central distribution hub of nerves of the trunk and limbs. When we talk about peripheral nerve injuries, we are talking about these large, long, anterior nerves, rather than the more superficial sensory nerves in the skin and muscle.

Many energy meridians correspond closely with the structure of the nerv-ous system. This is why the needling of points along nerve structures is an important factor in the effectiveness of acupuncture treatment. However, the closeness of these acupoints to many vulnerable peripheral nerves creates a risk of transient or more long-term injury.

Some of the more commonly used points where improper needling tech-nique can easily injure a peripheral nerve include:

- PC-6, PC-7, HT-3 – median nerve
- HT-7 – ulnar nerve
- LU-7 – radial nerve

- BL-60 – sural nerve
- GB-30 – sciatic nerve
- ST-36 – deep peroneal nerve
- TB-17 – great auricular nerve and, more deeply, facial nerve.

When we are using normal, ordinary needles, if we touch a nerve fibre the patient will have a strong reaction – even an electrical pulse sensation up and down the nerve. Other responses may include tingling or numbness. This may last several minutes or even a couple of hours. It is rare for this to result in long-term nerve damage, though it is possible if a point is stimulated too aggressively, too deeply or for too long, especially when using an electrical- or battery-powered stimulator.

Normally, the effects of nerve damage become apparent as inflammation sets in some hours or even a day after acupuncture treatment. The patient may experience tingling, numbness, diminished sensation, a feeling of heat or pain anywhere along the nerve pathway. In more extreme cases, there can be nerve palsy or paralysis, or even muscle atrophy. These symptoms are considered to be pathological changes from nerve damage.

Here we examine a few case studies of injuries reported in the literature.

Case study 1.5 Trigeminal nerve branch injury

A 50-year-old female was given acupuncture analgesia for a tooth extraction. ST-7 was needled too deeply, injuring the mandibular branch of the trigeminal nerve. This resulted in a flaccid masseter muscle, and a numb tongue unable to feel warmth. Five days of massage and warm compresses led to a full recovery (Gao et al 1993).

Case study 1.6 Trigeminal nerve branch injury

A 38-year-old female had been experiencing repeated throbbing pain on the left temple, for 2–5 minutes at a time, seven to 10 times a day for 2 years. Triggers for this pain included washing her face, brushing her teeth, blow-drying her hair and chewing. She consulted an acupuncturist, who needled ST-7, GB-8, LI-4 and Ex. Tai Yang. After 10 treatments the symptoms had much improved. During the 11th acupuncture treatment, the practitioner used a 2.5 cun needle in ST-7, inserting its entire length into the acupoint. The patient immediately felt burning pain at this site, and the practitioner removed the needle immediately. The patient had difficulty opening her mouth, and could

continued overpage

continued

> not chew, because of a muscle weakness on the left side. Treatment was
> stopped. After 3 days, the patient was gradually able to open her mouth,
> and several days later her chewing function gradually returned. This was
> clearly a case of excessive needling depth, injuring the mandibular branch of the
> trigeminal nerve which is motor to the chewing muscles. (Lun & Rong 1997).

Related acupoints

LI1-1 19, LI1-1 20
ST-1, ST-2, ST-3, ST-4, ST-5, ST-6, ST-7
SI-18, SI-19
GB-1, GB-2, GB-3
TB-17
Ren-24

Discussion of common injuries to facial and trigeminal nerves

Just below the ST-7 point there is a zygomatic branch from the facial nerve
and, more deeply, a branch of the trigeminal nerve called the mandibular
nerve. ST-7 is a very commonly used point in treating Bell's palsy, ear pain and
temporomandibular joint (TMJ) arthritis, as well as speech loss after stroke, so
practitioners must think about the proximity of two major cranial nerves
whenever we are needling the face. Most of the above-listed points are in this
same area.

The trigeminal is the fifth cranial nerve, which comes from the pons, in the
brain, and expands to form the semilunar ganglion, then branches out further
into the ophthalmic, maxillary and mandibular nerves. The mandibular is the
biggest nerve of the three, and dominates motor functions of the masseter
muscle, as well as sensations of the lower teeth, gums, the front two-thirds of
the tongue and the bottom of the mouth and the skin of the lower cheek. If
this nerve is injured, the patient will mainly experience paralysis of the muscles involved in chewing, and reduction in sensation of pain and temperature
in the tongue. In severe cases, sensation can disappear entirely.

The facial nerve is the seventh cranial nerve, also beginning in the pons,
starting at the base of the skull, going into the parotid gland, then branching
into 5 sections that dominate motor functions of the muscles, which create
expression in the face. It also affects motor function in the platysma, the

posterior belly of the digastric muscle, and the stylohyoid muscle. An injury to the facial nerve results in symptoms such as the disappearance of wrinkles in part of the forehead, and of the nasolabial sulcus – the skin fold that commonly runs from the nostrils to the corner of the mouth. Also, there may be a twisting of the mouth toward the uninjured side. The patient will probably be unable to close the eyelid on the injured side.

When the points listed above are needled, especially ST-7, practitioners have to be gentle and always keep the anatomy of these nerves in mind to avoid injury, especially when using electrical stimulation. It is also advisable, when using electrical stimulation, to begin at the lowest setting and increase the stimulation only in small, slow increments.

In China, there have been many reports of injury to these nerves caused by injection of Chinese or Western medications, such as cortisone, into ST-7 and other acupoints. This is used in treatment for Bell's palsy, among other conditions that cause paralysis in the face. The danger with this procedure is that a volume of fluid can put excessive pressure on the nerves. Damage can also result if the pH of the medication used is too acidic or alkaline. Until recently, this procedure was not commonly performed by practitioners in most Western countries, unless they were medical doctors or otherwise authorised to give injections, but point injection is making its way into the scope of practice of trained acupuncturists in some jurisdictions.

Case study 1.7 Median nerve neuropathy

In a rare and unusual accident, a needle in either PC-6 or PC-7 was broken in the patient's carpal tunnel, causing an inflammation of the median nerve. Hot compresses and physiotherapy were administered for relief (Peuker & Gronemeyer 2001).

Case study 1.8 Median nerve injury

A male patient arrived for acupuncture treatment for a stomach problem. When the practitioner worked on PC-6, the patient felt an 'electric shock' along the arm. The acupuncturist misread this symptom, thinking it came from the de qi energy reaction and increased the stimulation of the point. This resulted in a burning sensation along the patient's median nerve. After treatment, the patient's wrist felt numb, and movement in the wrist and thumb was impaired (Jiang 1988).

Case study 1.9 Median nerve injury

The author reported two cases of injury, both of which were incurred while working on PC-6. The practitioner used 1.5 cun needles on this point, inserting them into the tissue to a depth of 1.2 cun, right through the nerve. He continued to apply vigorous stimulation, continuing for 15 minutes. After this treatment, one patient experienced a flexion of the fingers and was unable to straighten them. The practitioner began moxibustion and massage on the wrist, observing the patient for 30 minutes. The patient's hand function returned to normal.

The second patient also experienced flexion, as well as pain and a loss of temperature sensation in the fingers. Moxa treatment, massage and exercises were prescribed, and a week later the patient had recovered fully. The author's analysis of these two cases cites an injury to the median nerve as the cause of the hand muscle contraction. In my opinion, the depth of needling in these two cases was excessive; in an average-sized person a maximum penetration of less than 1.25 cm (half inch) is indicated (Wang 1991).

Related acupoints

HT-3
PC-3, PC-4, PC-5, PC-6, PC-7
Ex. Er Bai, Ex. Bi Zhong

Discussion of injury to median nerves

The median nerve runs along the middle of the arm and forearm to the hand, and lies between the ulnar and the musculocutaneous and radial nerves. It follows the pericardium meridian in the forearm, close to the wrist. As the nerve is close to the surface, care must be taken not to needle the above points too deeply (Fig. 1.3). If this nerve is touched, the patient will feel a severe electrical sensation and you must withdraw the needle a bit. If aggressive stimulation is performed, the nerve can be seriously injured, causing both sensory and motor disorders in the thumb and next two fingers: numbness, burning pain, decreased touch and temperature sensations, inability to flex the wrist and the first three fingers, and inability to pronate the wrist and perform opposition with the thumb ('monkey hand').

Mild cases can be treated with massage, warming with a moxa stick, and making warm wet compresses and a tea of the following herbs to increase circulation and speed recovery.

Healing nerve preparation:

- 12 grams Bai Shao Yao (white peony)
- 6 grams Chuan Xiong (ligusticum)

- 6 grams Qiang Huo (notopterygium)
- 9 grams Sang Zhi (mulberry twig)
- 15 grams Ji Xue Teng (milettia)

Mix one package of herbs with about five cups of water; cook down to two cups of water; drink one cup in the morning, another in the late afternoon. Repeat daily for 1–2 weeks. You can also use Zheng Gu Shui tincture mixed with hot water for a compress, applied 10–15 minutes once a day.

Gentle, shallow needling will prevent injury to the median nerve. Ask the patient to report any sensations during treatment and respond accordingly. If the patient complains of feeling a strong electrical pulse, withdraw the needle 1–2 mm and the sensation should subside.

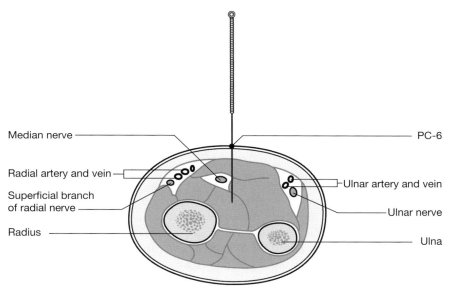

Figure 1.3 Correct needle position in PC-6. When needling PC-6, the needle should go along the ulnar side of the median nerve, rather than the radial side, to avoid puncturing the nerve. If the median nerve is touched, the patient will feel a strong electrical sensation.

Case study 1.10 Radial nerve injury

A 52-year-old female complaining of headaches came for acupuncture. The practitioner treated several points including LU-7. After the second treatment, the patient felt pain and numbness on the radial side of the left wrist, radiating from the treatment site up to the elbow. After a week, during which she was given massage and moxa treatment, the numbness and pain were gone (Shen 1983).

Case study 1.11 Radial nerve injury

In this case, a male, 40 years of age, requested treatment for hepatitis. The acupuncturist selected several points including LU-7. On stimulation of the needle at that point, the patient experienced a sensation similar to electric shock, followed by numbness and tingling, from the point on the wrist down to the thumb and up the arm to the elbow. Following treatment, an examination found the patient had difficulty in flexing his thumb and his hand. Normal skin sensation in the webbing between the thumb and index finger was also reduced. It took a month of physiotherapy, applications of heat and vitamin B supplements before the patient's functioning and sensation were close to normal (Cheng et al 1963).

Related acupoints

LU-5, LU-6, LU-7, LU-8, LU-9, LU-10
LI-4, LI-5, LI-6, LI-7, LI-10, LI-11
TB-5, TB-6, TB-7
SI-9

Discussion of injury to radial nerve

The radial nerve runs from the upper arm down into the hand (Fig. 1.4). At the upper end, it lies slightly to the outer side of the radial artery, tucked under the supinator longus. Just above the elbow, it separates into two branches, one of which is deep (internal); the other more external or shallow branch is closer to the forearm. When the above points, all of which are fairly close to the wrist, are needled too deeply or aggressively, sensory symptoms include: numbness, burning pain and decreased sensations of touch and temperature. Other symptoms may be a sensation of an electrical pulse radiating to the dorsal side of the thumb and index finger.

Damage to motor functions is evident when the patient is unable to supinate the wrist and extend the wrist and all fingers – a condition known as 'wrist-drop'. In a severe case, the patient will be unable to lift the thumb while the rest of the hand is flat on a table. Full recovery is usual, under the proper care. More specific information on treating peripheral nerve injuries is given elsewhere in this section, but, in general, the sooner treatment (massage, compresses, etc.) is begun – preferably within 24 hours – the more likely it is that the symptoms will disappear quickly. If there is little or no improvement after 2 weeks of treatment of the injury, the patient should be referred to a neurologist.

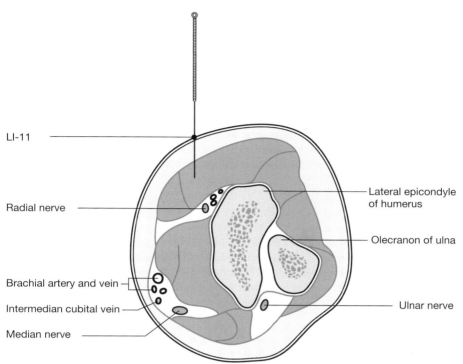

Figure 1.4 Correct needle depth in LI-11. Excessive needle depth in LI-11 will injure the radial nerve, causing an electrical shock sensation in the forearm and hand.

Case study 1.12 Ulnar nerve injury

The patient was a 45-year-old male, whose complaint was insomnia. The acupuncturist employed the HT-7 point, placing the needle in an oblique direction towards LU-9, with strong stimulation. This was painful for the patient, who asked that the needle be removed. He felt very tired after the treatment and had to sit in the waiting room for an hour until he recovered his energy. After treatment, he experienced numbness in the fingers and the palm of his hand, though motor function was not affected. After 3 days the numbness had worn off in all but the last two fingers. Four more acupuncture treatments, over the course of a month, relieved the remaining numbness (Gao et al 1993).

Related acupoints

HT-1, HT-2, HT-4, HT-5, HT-6, HT-7
SI-6, SI-8

Discussion of injury to ulnar nerve

The ulnar nerve is the major motor nerve of the hand and the ulnar side of the forearm (flexor muscles). It also supplies sensation to the ulnar side of the forearm (Fig. 1.5). The ulnar nerve travels along the inner side of the arm, and branches off into the muscles and skin of the forearm and hand. At its upper end, it lies to the inner side of the axillary artery, then runs obliquely across the internal head of the triceps. At the elbow it passes behind the medial condyle (the funny bone!) and passes into the forearm to the pisiform bone of the wrist.

The nerve is especially shallow under SI-8 and HT-7. Signs of sensory damage are numbness, pain, and decreased touch and temperature sensations. Damage to motor functions is evident in weakness of elbow flexion, inability to move the fourth and fifth fingers (interossei muscle palsy), inability to flex the thumb, and weakness in the minor thenar eminence. If the nerve is seriously injured causing muscular atrophy and poor circulation, the fourth and fifth fingers remain slightly curved. In more serious injuries, the muscles between the intermetarcarpal bones can atrophy, resulting in a clawed hand. Usually the nerve is merely touched, creating an electrical sensation, and recovery is complete within 2 days to 1 week.

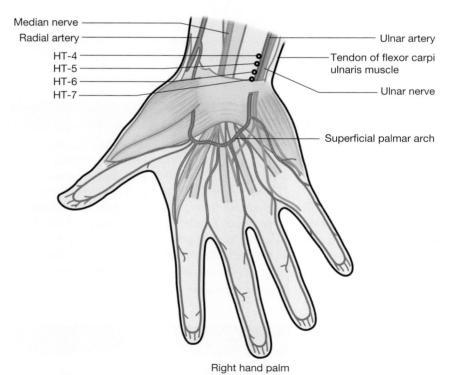

Right hand palm

Figure 1.5 Correct needling position in HT-4 to HT-7. Shallow needling, angled toward the radial side of the wrist, will avoid puncture of the ulnar nerve.

All the motor functions of the hand are dominated by the ulnar nerve, with the exception of a small group: the short abductor muscle and short flexor muscle of the thumb, the opposing muscle of the thumb, and the first and second lumbrical muscles. Motor functions in these muscles are controlled by the medial nerve. The ulnar nerve also controls sensory function in the ulnar side of the hand; the rest of the hand's sensation comes from the medial nerve. Information about prevention and treatment of injuries is included in the general discussion of peripheral nerve damage.

Case study 1.13 Deep peroneal nerve palsy

A 1-year-old boy was being treated for acute tuberculosis, with a combination of Western medicine, traditional Chinese medicine and acupuncture treatments. ST-36 was one of the points used. Two days after the acupuncture treatment, the child was found to have drop-foot – a weakness in the right foot and a swollen ankle joint. Physiotherapy, massage, Vitamin B and acupuncture treatments gradually resolved these effects (Cheng et al 1963).

Case study 1.14 Deep peroneal nerve palsy

Another case of drop-foot was caused by needling of GB-34, which reaches the common peroneal nerve where the deep peroneal nerve splits off from it. The bladder meridian points listed below are also close to the common peroneal and tibial nerves, and are therefore vulnerable to trauma from needles inserted too deeply or stimulated too strongly (Peuker & Gronemeyer 2001).

Case study 1.15 Common peroneal nerve injury

The patient was a 29-year-old male who for 2 weeks had been having lower back pain and difficulty in walking. Acupuncture treatment involved the use of a 1 cun needle in GB-34, with strong thrusting and lifting. The patient felt electrical sensations shooting down his entire leg to the foot. Then an injection of a mixture of dang gui (dong quai) and tian ma (gastrodia) was administered into the same point. After the injection, the patient felt pain, numbness and weakness in the leg, which affected his ability to walk. An injury of the common peroneal nerve was diagnosed.

Moxa treatment was given for the injury, twice a day for 15 minutes. The patient was fully recovered a week later (Xia 1993).

Related acupoints (common peroneal and deep peroneal nerve)
ST-36, ST-37, ST-38, ST-39, ST-41
GB-34
BL-38, BL-39
Ex. Lan Wei Xu (Appendix point)

Discussion of injury to peroneal nerves

The common peroneal nerve is a branch of the sciatic nerve that travels down the lateral leg to the lateral side of the popliteal fossa behind the biceps femoris tendon to the neck of the fibula (GB-34). Here it divides into shallow and deep branches; the deep branch travels under the anterior tibialis muscle to the dorsum of the foot (Fig. 1.6). It dominates the anterior leg muscles and dorsal muscles of the foot. Although the peroneal nerve runs deeply, there are many acupuncture points located along it. That is why reports of deep peroneal nerve injury associated with acupuncture are so common.

Sensory injury leads to numbness on the lateral side of the front of the leg and the top of the foot. Motor injury causes weakness of the leg, foot-drop (inability to dorsiflex the foot and toes), ankle swelling and possibly muscular atrophy. For information on treatment modalities, see 'What to do in case of peripheral nerve injury', later in this chapter. Prevent deep peroneal nerve injuries by avoiding deep insertion and excessive stimulation to obtain de qi.

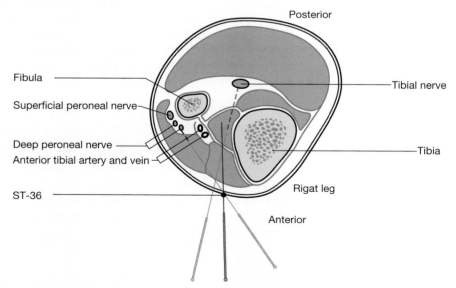

Figure 1.6 Correct and incorrect angles of needling in ST-36. The needle should be aimed between the tibial and peroneal bones to avoid hitting the nearby nerves. Placement should not be too deep.

Related acupoints (tibial nerves)

SP-6, SP-7, SP-8, SP-9
BL1-1 40, BL-55, BL-56, BL-57
KI-3, KI-4, KI-5, KI-6, KI-7, KI-8, KI-9
LIV-7, LIV-8

Discussion of injury to tibial nerve

Considering the number of points in close proximity to the tibial nerve, it is somewhat surprising not to find case studies of related injuries in the medical literature. Perhaps this is because these injuries are rarely, if ever, severe. However, there are a number of anecdotal reports.

The tibial nerve is the extension of the main trunk of the sciatic nerve; it runs along the median line of the popliteal fossa of the leg (Fig. 1.7). It runs behind the triceps muscle of the calf, along the posterior tibial artery, then next to the ankle joint to the bottom of the foot. This nerve dominates motor and sensory function of the calf muscle and the sole of the foot. If the tibial nerve is injured the foot and toes will be incapable of plantar flexion. In addition, adduction and inversion of the foot are impaired. The patient will be unable to stand or walk on the toes. Severe cases result in a 'hook' foot, in which the anterolateral muscle of the leg contracts extremely, causing the foot to be twisted toward the outside of the body. Sensory damage includes numbness, or loss of sensation or temperature sensitivity in the sole and lateral edge of the foot. In a severe injury that has not been properly treated, muscle atrophy and contraction will eventually draw the foot into a crabbed shape like a horse's hoof.

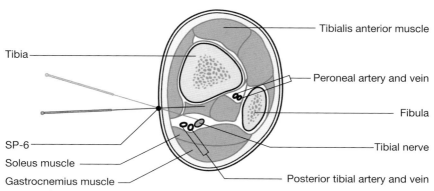

Figure 1.7 Correct angle of needling in SP-6. To avoid puncturing the tibial nerve, the needle should be aimed along the back edge of the tibial bone rather than into the calf muscle.

What to do in case of peripheral nerve injury

If the patient feels strong nerve pain or electrical sensation, withdraw the needle slightly and change the angle of penetration. If the patient has a more serious reaction, and sensation is intolerable even after withdrawal and adjustment of the needle, remove the needle and do not continue to work on this point.

You can use very gentle massage, moxa and a warm compress. If the patient is still experiencing discomfort the next day, you may recommend a consultation with a physiotherapist.

Supplements of Vitamin B complex will assist in recovery of nerves. For information on therapeutic dosages of vitamins, you might want to consult a pharmacist or naturopathic physician.

If motor function is only slightly impaired, encourage the patient to exercise the affected part gently. After 2 weeks, if symptoms haven't improved, refer the patient to a physician, who might then recommend a consultation with a specialist.

Prevention of peripheral nerve injury

When we work on points along meridians that run just over nerve structures, we must familiarise ourselves with these structures and always bear in mind the locations and depths of nearby nerves when preparing to insert needles.

When the needle feels resistance, and you sense that the tissue it is touching is pliable but tough, the tip of the needle is touching the branch of a nerve. You will also be getting feedback from the patient at this point! Back the needle off – at least 2 mm. After that, when you are stimulating the needles, be particularly gentle.

Excessive depth of needling is the major cause of peripheral nerve damage, so if you are not absolutely sure of the depth of the nerve trunk or branch, check before you treat. It's better to place a needle slightly too shallow than too deep.

When using electric acupuncture to work on points close to nerves, you must be extremely careful not to increase the level of stimulation too quickly. Start slowly, ask the patient for feedback, and increase in small, slow increments to allow the patient's body to adjust to each level of stimulation. Electrical stimulation of nerves can cause extreme discomfort to the patient.

INTERCOSTAL BLOOD VESSEL INJURY

There is a common belief that the intercostal blood vessels are not at serious risk of injury, because they are small, almost invisible from the outside of the body, and therefore hard to puncture. However this is a misconception. Several chest points (LIV-13, LIV-14, GB-22, GB-24) and back shu points are used frequently – even daily – in practice, and the more commonly used points of course have a higher rate of injury associated with them than those that are rarely employed. Puncture of an intercostal vessel can cause death, so it is important to know how to avoid such injuries.

A common question on examinations gives us a hint of the anatomical knowledge necessary in this case:

'When needling chest points, is it safest to place the needle tip:

a. towards the lower border of the upper rib
b. towards the upper border of the lower rib
c. precisely between the ribs.'

The answer, as you should know, is 'c', because of the location of the related blood vessels.

A brief review of the anatomy of intercostal vessels is in order here. Beginning on the front of the body, the arch of the aorta branches into the right and left subclavian arteries. For this discussion we follow the left branch, which divides into four major vessels. One of these is the internal thoracic artery, which itself splits into a number of vessels, including the anterior intercostal arteries. These supply the six upper intercostal spaces. Each intercostal artery forms two smaller branches; one lies along the lower edge of the rib above, and the other runs close to the upper edge of the rib below.

Another branch of the internal thoracic artery is the musculophrenic artery, which splits into anterior arteries that correspond with the lower five intercostal spaces. These also run along the upper and lower edges of the ribs. Therefore a needle that is placed precisely in the centre of the intercostal space will miss these vessels.

Moving now to the back of the body, the thoracic aorta divides into vessels that supply blood to various organs, and into a parietal branch that splits into four vessels. Two of these – the posterior intercostal artery and the subcostal artery – are relevant to this discussion.

The intercostal arteries come out of the back of the aorta and supply the third to 11th intercostal spaces (Fig. 1.8). Like the anterior arteries, they branch into upper and lower sections. But they are placed differently; the upper branch is nestled into the groove in the inside lower border of the rib. Above the artery is a vein, and below it is a nerve, except in the upper intercostal spaces where the nerve is above the artery. The lower branch lies on the upper border of the lower rib. The upper and lower branches meet at the internal thoracic artery and musculophrenic artery.

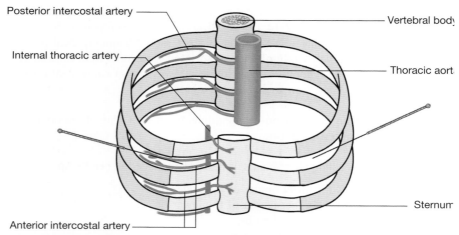

Posterior intercostal artery

Internal thoracic artery

Vertebral body

Thoracic aort

Sternum

Anterior intercostal artery

Figure 1.8 Arteries that serve the thoracic wall. The needle is shown entering the intercostal space at the correct angle, which is oblique in relation to the skin surface.

The subcostal artery, which comes from the parietal branch, runs along the lower border of the last rib – the 12th intercostal space.

Moving back up the body for a moment, the first and second intercostal spaces on the back are supplied by superior intercostal arteries; these are a branch of the costocervical trunk, which is a branch of the subclavian artery. The subclavian, as we saw above, arises from the arch of the aorta.

Why do acupuncturists need to understand this level of detail? First, although the intercostal vessels themselves are fairly small, they are close to the major power centre of circulation: the aorta. So the blood pressure is high and bleeding may be severe if nearby vessels are punctured. Secondly, the information about the way the intercostal vessels run along the ribs helps us understand the importance of needling as precisely as we can in the space between the ribs –as far away from veins and arteries as possible.

Case study 1.16

An adult male experienced bloating and abdominal discomfort after meals and a diminishing appetite. His condition worsened over the course of 6 months, and he was eventually diagnosed with hepatitis.

Early one afternoon, he was given acupuncture to relieve these symptoms. During the treatment, the patient suddenly began to cough. Although the needles were removed, the man developed shortness of breath, and severe abdominal pain that was aggravated by lying on his right side, and vomiting. Later that evening he was admitted to hospital; his pulse was 140, and his blood pressure so weak as to be almost inaudible. The man's abdomen was swollen, rigid and tender to the touch. Marks of the acupuncture needles were still evident on both sides of the chest.

Physicians performed abdominal paracentesis, and withdrew fluids and blood from the abdominal cavity. Intravenous glucose and dextran were administered immediately, and the patient injected with adrenaline (epinephrine) and given oxygen. During preparations for a blood transfusion and surgery, the patient suffered cardiac and pulmonary arrest, and died. Autopsy found 2700 ml of blood in the man's abdominal cavity, and a 4 × 14 cm retroperitoneal haematoma close to the lower border of the right 10th rib. This matched the entry point of a needle at LIV-13. The pathologist reported that an acupuncture needle had ruptured an intercostal artery, resulting in severe bleeding into the abdominal cavity and death by shock (Shao 1977).

Related acupoints

All SP, ST, KI, PC, GB, LIV, BL and Ren points over the ribcage

Discussion of intercostal vessel injury

Acupuncture practitioners are seeing more and more people with shingles or intercostal neuralgia who are seeking treatment on their own, or being referred by their physicians. Acupuncture is very effective in these cases. In traditional Chinese medicine theory, many symptoms are attributed to stagnation in the Liver and Gall Bladder meridians, and the most common and useful points for removing these energy blockages are located over the ribcage.

When a needle hits an intercostal vessel, the blood can flow in one of two directions. If the puncture is deep enough, there will be bleeding into either the thoracic or abdominal cavity, resulting in haemorrhagic pleurisy or haemorrhagic peritonitis. Severe blood loss can lead to shock and even death; a case such as the one cited above is uncommon, but is a useful reminder to maintain sharp vigilance even when using points we employ every day.

If the wound has not penetrated the abdominal or pulmonary cavities, the blood can pool under or within muscle or soft tissue, forming a haematoma, or flow out when the needle is removed. This is a less serious situation than the first, because we can at least see that there is something wrong. Internal bleeding may be undetectable until it becomes life threatening.

What to do in case of intercostal vessel injury

Appropriate first aid treatment varies, depending on the severity of the injury. In a mild puncture, where a small amount of blood is leaking or spurting from the needle site, applying pressure to the wound with a sterile cotton ball for a few minutes should stop the bleeding. If bruising or a small haematoma appears, a cold compress should be used several times a day for a couple of days. After that, a heating pad will help the body reabsorb the blood. Whether cold or warm, the compress should be used for 15–20 minutes at a time. In a week to 10 days, the bruising or haematoma should be fully dispersed.

The patient should not be exhibiting any other symptoms if the injury is minor. However, if the patient is pale, develops rapid and shallow breathing, the pulse becomes weak and fast or blood pressure drops, we should suspect internal bleeding, which must be treated as an emergency to prevent the patient from going into shock. An ambulance should be called immediately to transport the patient to hospital for treatment.

Prevention of intercostal vessel injury

When treating points in the intercostal spaces, it is safest to needle at an oblique angle – about 45° relative to the surface of the thorax – toward the outside of the body. On points that are closer to the lateral edges of the thorax, the angle should be even flatter – more like 15–25°. The depth of insertion should be very shallow, especially when the patient is thin. Insertion should be done very slowly, and stimulation must be gentle.

Do not assume that the fatty tissue of a woman's breast gives much protection from a puncture wound. Breast tissue is richly supplied with blood vessels, and there are reports in the literature of intercostal vessels beneath the breasts being pierced by improperly placed acupuncture needles.

Most importantly, ensure that the needle is inserted precisely in the middle of the space between the ribs to avoid contacting the vessels, as is outlined in the anatomy section above (Fig. 1.9). Be sure that the tip of the needle is pointing parallel to the line of the rib, and not up or down towards either rib.

ARTERIAL PUNCTURE

In the literature, bleeding (minor or major) from blood vessel punctures is listed among the most common acupuncture accidents.

Acupuncture injury can occur to arteries, veins or capillaries. Because arterial blood is under higher pressure, blood loss will be more significant than in the case of punctures to the other vessels. That is why our discussion here will focus on arteries.

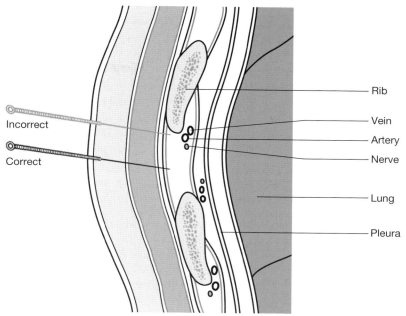

Incorrect

Correct

Rib

Vein

Artery

Nerve

Lung

Pleura

Figure 1.9 Cutaway view of intercostal vessel showing incorrect and correct needle placement. (Refer to Figure 1.8 for correct angle of insertion, which should be oblique to the skin.)

However, this does not mean practitioners should forget about veins and capillaries when we are plotting our treatment points. These, too, can be pierced through careless technique. The sections on preventing and treating punctures are applicable to all vessels.

Case study 1.17

A 64-year-old male was requesting acupuncture for chest congestion and pain in the costal regions of both sides, and aching in both arms. The acupuncturist chose LIV-14, SI-15, LI-4 and Ex. Tai Yang points. The patient was kept in a sitting position for treatment. On the last point, LIV-14, the practitioner used a 1.5 cun needle. One minute after insertion of the needle, the patient began shouting for the treatment to stop, and lay down on the table, grabbing his chest. He quickly lost consciousness, and developed sweating and urinary incontinence. All needles were immediately removed. In an attempt to resuscitate the patient, Du-26 was needled and CPR performed for 15 minutes, but the man died. An autopsy found an acupuncture hole 2.7 cm. toward the midline, measuring from the patient's left nipple, in a diagonal direction through the muscle, into the mediastinum and finally breaking into the thoracic aorta. There were 400 ml of blood in the pericardial cavity; pressure from the volume of liquid had stopped the man's heart.

continued overpage

continued

> The reviewer's analysis of this case was that the acupuncturist had been extremely incompetent in his choice of points. He should have placed the needle in the sixth intercostal space, below the left nipple. Instead, he inserted it between KI-22 and KI-23 – clearly a mistake. In addition, the angle and depth were wrong. Cause of death was cardiac arrest (Zhu 1990).

Discussion of arterial puncture

Points listed in Table 1.1 are chosen because they are either directly under, or close to an artery. These vessels, therefore, are vulnerable to puncture if needle depth or direction is wrong. This is not an exhaustive list; the chart covers the most likely injury sites, and includes points that have been collected from case reports of injuries. In some cases, a needle going through a given point can pierce different arteries, depending on the angle of insertion. This is why some points appear in more than one category.

For the sake of conciseness and clarity, the table names only the major arterial branches in question, unless an acupoint is directly on one of the smaller ends of a vessel. Bear in mind that many of the arteries have a corresponding vein nearby.

The result of an arterial puncture can range from minor, when only a small vessel such as a capillary is involved, to quite serious, leading to bleeding, haematoma or false traumatic aneurysm. Although faulty technique is generally the cause of the accident, its effects may be exacerbated by factors related to the patient's health. The person may have a very low blood platelet count. Haemophilia is a serious risk factor. A liver with advanced disease may not produce enough globulin to ensure sufficient clotting. Blood-thinning medications will also influence the likelihood of bleeding. Also, some patients have sclerosis of the blood vessels, impairing the elasticity of the walls and making them more brittle, and therefore vulnerable.

A tiny amount of bleeding is a common occurrence in acupuncture practice. But a needle injury to an artery can be fatal. In one case, a patient's aorta was ruptured by a needle in LIV-14. In another, a practitioner treating LIV-13 punctured an intercostal artery, resulting in intraperitoneal haemorrhage, shock and death.

What to do in case of arterial puncture

Because the outer layers of arteries are rich in nerve endings, an injury to this structure will be painful to the patient. Unlike a nerve puncture, which sends an electrical pulse along the body, or a muscle and ligament tear, which causes

Table 1.1 Artery-related acupoints most commonly used

Artery and/or branch	Related acupoints
Arch of the aorta	Ren-22 (Fig. 1.11)
Common carotid artery	ST-9 (Fig. 1.10), ST-10, ST-11, LI-18
Internal carotid artery	SI-17
Transverse cervical artery	ST-12
Facial artery	LI-19, LI-20, ST-5
Transverse facial artery	ST-7
Superficial temporal artery	SI-19, TB-21, GB-2
Inferior thyroid artery	Ren-22
Posterior auricular artery	SI-16
Occipital artery	SI-16
Subclavian artery	ST-11, ST-12
Lateral thoracic artery	GB-22
Intercostal arteries	GB-22, LIV-13, LIV-14
Axillary artery	HT-1
Brachial artery	PC-3
Radial artery	LU-6, LU-8, LU-9
Ulnar artery	HT-4, HT-5, HT-6, HT-7
Superior ulnar collateral artery	HT-2
Radial recurrent artery	LU-5, LI-10
Superficial palmar arch	PC-8
Deep palmar arch	LI-4
Inferior epigastric artery	ST-30, LIV-12
Femoral artery	SP-10, SP-11, SP-12, SP-13, LIV-9, LIV-11, LIV-12
Deep femoral artery	LIV-11
Medial femoral circumflex artery	LIV-10
Popliteal artery	BL-40
Medial superior genicular artery	KI-10
Lateral inferior genicular artery	GB-34
Anterior tibial artery	ST-36, GB-39
Posterior tibial artery	KI-3
Dorsal artery of foot	ST-42

a deep, heavy ache, the pain from a punctured artery is sharp and localised. It can last from several seconds to several days.

The obvious sign of a puncture is bleeding, which may spurt or seep from the wound, or collect under the skin as a bruise or haematoma. A haematoma can impede circulation, which would be evident in coldness and pallor of the skin around the area. Severe complications of arterial puncture include traumatic aneurysm, haemathorax or haemorrhagic peritonitis, depending on the site of the wound.

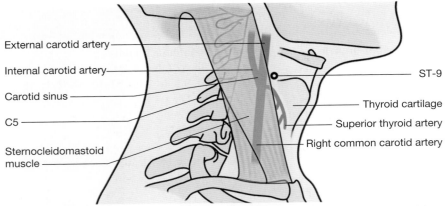

Figure 1.10 Correct location of ST-9. When needling ST-9, the needle should be placed in front of the sternocleidomastoid muscle to avoid puncturing the carotid artery.

A patient who is very sensitive, or who is losing a quantity of blood, may exhibit one or more signs of shock: lightheadedness or dizziness, nervousness, sweating, facial pallor, rapid, shallow breathing or a drop in blood pressure.

If blood seeps from the acupoint when you withdraw the needle, use a sterile cotton ball to press gently on the point for a minute or two, until the bleeding stops. If the patient is taking anticoagulant medications such as warfarin, you will need to press longer; depending on the individual's coagulation time, this could be 3 more minutes.

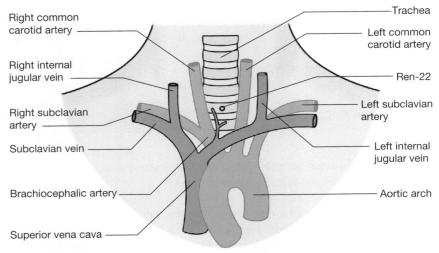

Figure 1.11 Vessels surrounding Ren-22. The correct depth of penetration in this point is 0.2 cun at perpendicular, then change the angle of needle to oblique, placing less than 1 cun behind the sternum. This will avoid puncturing many large vessels.

If you do not see any blood seeping from the hole, but it is collecting under the skin and forming a small haematoma, first press with a cotton ball to stop the bleeding, then massage the area to disperse the haematoma. If you can feel a swelling more deeply in the tissues, ask the patient to go home and apply ice packs to the area two or three times a day for 2 days, for 15–20 minutes each time, to reduce the swelling. On the 3rd day, heat should be applied to help disperse the collected blood.

During acupuncture treatment, if a larger vessel has been punctured, whether or not blood is spurting out or pooling under the skin, apply a pressure bandage over the wound and a tourniquet between it and the heart. Call for emergency assistance. It is extremely rare for this to occur, but the patient may need to be treated for shock, or require a blood transfusion or even surgery. If you suspect you've punctured one of the larger vessels, don't take chances. Call an ambulance immediately. The potential consequences to the patient are more important than the practitioner's possible embarrassment.

Prevention of arterial puncture

When seeing patients for the first time, always ask whether they have any blood-related problems such as coagulation disorders, or take any anticoagulant medications. Many people take a daily prophylactic dose of baby aspirin. This is not a problem. However, aspirin taken in large quantities as a blood thinner is in the same category as other anticoagulant medications. If this is the case, avoid treating any points that are close to larger blood vessels, many of which are listed in Table 1.1. When treating patients who take anticoagulants, even when using only the safest points, it is recommended that a cotton ball is used to press on each point for a few seconds just after withdrawing each needle. The patient should also be observed while preparing to leave the clinic, to watch for any bleeding.

Detailed knowledge of anatomy is crucial when treating points over medium- or large-sized blood vessels. It is a good idea to consult textbooks before placing needles, until you have enough clinical experience to be completely familiar with the surface projections of major vessels. Sometimes newer practitioners will use a clean, non-toxic eyebrow pencil to mark the geography of the vessels, especially the carotid, aorta, intercostal and femoral arteries, before placing needles in their vicinity. In China, acupuncturists still resort to old-fashioned but effective markers as mercurochrome or gentian violet, which offer the added benefit of being antiseptics.

As always, when working around vulnerable areas, watch the depth and direction of insertion, and ensure stimulation is gentle.

Because the wall of the artery is made of many elastic fibres, when the needle touches the arterial wall you will feel a resistance to the needle that is slightly tougher than that from the skin and subcutaneous tissue. This indicates it is time to back off the needle.

Another signal is that when a needle is on or even close to an artery you will be able to see a slight pulsation as it moves with the arterial action. My technique when treating these sensitive points is to insert the needle into the subcutaneous tissue, just short of the depth recommended in the texts, then remove my hand and observe whether there is any movement. If not, the needle can be pushed slightly further. Again, I remove my hand and observe. Sometimes I will do this as many as three times to allow the needle to 'speak' to me. If the needle is pulsing, it should be backed off, whether or not de qi has been reached. If I have not sensed de qi, I will leave the needle there while I work on the other treatment points. Then I return to this point, and gently rotate the needle to obtain de qi. It is important to remember that de qi is not necessarily achieved by more depth.

When a large vessel has been punctured, it will soon become obvious, as severe symptoms such as those listed above will appear. However, an injury to a small vessel or capillary may not be evident until the needles are removed at the end of the treatment. So, even when the whole treatment has gone smoothly, the practitioner cannot be absolutely certain that there has been no injury until all needles are removed – in essence, 'uncorking' all the holes – and there are no signs of bleeding or haematoma. Special techniques for purging excess Heat, which may involve the loss of a drop or two of blood, do not fall into this category.

In this section we have covered information about blood vessel injuries in general; now we will examine some specific ones that have special features.

TRAUMATIC ANEURYSM

An aneurysm is a bulge in the wall of an artery (Fig. 1.12). The bulge generally occurs in a weak spot in the arterial wall. Many of these result from a congeni-

Figure 1.12 Traumatic aneurysm. A traumatic aneurysm, shown on the left, is also called a false aneurysm. It is caused by an injury, including that from an acupuncture needle. The illustration on the right is a 'true' aneurysm, the bulging that results from a weakness in the vessel's wall.

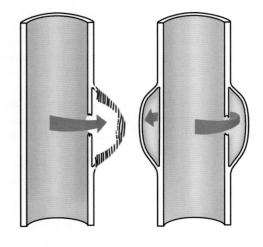

A traumatic (false) aneurysm   A true aneurysm

tal weakness or arteriosclerosis; others come from injuries caused by stab or gun-shot wounds, or from bacterial or fungal infections in the wall of the artery. Acupuncture is one of the unusual but possible sources of a traumatic aneurysm.

Case study 1.18

A 61-year-old woman sought medical treatment for a pulsating mass that had been enlarging in her left thigh for 4 months. Approximately 2 months before the lump first appeared, she had received one acupuncture treatment to relieve pain from osteoarthritis in her knees. During this treatment, the practitioner had placed multiple needles around the woman's left knee and along the inner thigh. The patient complained of sharp pains at some of the needle sites; after the needles were removed the pain disappeared.

Four months later, while the woman was sitting in a chair, she felt a sudden shooting pain from her left thigh to the lower leg.

Though the pain went away on its own, a large, deep bruise appeared in the area several days later. Over the following months the woman's left thigh continued to swell and she eventually presented herself at a medical clinic.

An examination and an MRI scan revealed a pulsating mass, 10 × 10 cm. in size, on the lower part of the woman's left inner thigh. In surgery, there was a clear perforation of the popliteal artery, corresponding with the sac of the aneurysm. A large clot was removed and the lesion was repaired. The surgery was successful; the patient was discharged after 5 days in hospital and recovered completely (Kao & Chang 2002).

Related acupoints

Refer to Table 1.1. Any of the medium- or large-sized vessels can receive an injury that results in an aneurysm; the very small vessels would not be subject to this, as they would form only a dead-end haematoma.

Discussion of traumatic aneurysm

When an acupuncture needle injures an artery or one of its branches it causes internal bleeding; the surrounding tissue, including blood platelets and fibrin, collects in a mass around the wound. As arterial blood continues to flow into the bulge, the mass grows and its wall thickens. The pulsing pressure of arterial blood in this mass will be palpable, and can be heard through a stethoscope.

The whole process can take several weeks, or even up to a year to develop before ischaemic and pressure symptoms cause the patient to see a physician.

The mass, which can be deeply buried under thick muscles, may be mistaken for an abscess or infection; if a blood sample is drawn from the bulge, the problem can be easily misdiagnosed as a regular, isolated haematoma from a sports injury, for example. If the patient happens to mention to the doctor that this problem has developed after acupuncture in the area, it will be a useful clue to correct diagnosis.

Any aneurysm can be ruptured or become infected. These factors further complicate accurate diagnosis and treatment.

The literature on acupuncture-related accidents relates cases of aneurysm in the following vessels: the common carotid artery, the superior gluteal artery, the costocervical artery, the popliteal artery and the abdominal aorta. All of these patients recovered after surgery to repair the damaged artery.

What to do in case of traumatic aneurysm

A patient who has suffered a traumatic aneurysm may complain of a progressively growing, pulsating lump that is tender or painful to the touch. There may also be functional problems from the lack of circulation to a particular area; for instance, if there is damage to the popliteal artery the patient may have trouble walking.

Ultrasound usually clearly reveals the location and size of an aneurysm; if the mass is particularly deep, or obscured by other tissue, a CT or MRI scan may be necessary. A history of acupuncture in the affected area will also inform the diagnostic process. Surgery is the most likely course of action. This may involve excising the mass, and repairing the injury to the arterial wall, by performing either an end-to-end anastomosis, or inserting an arterial graft using an artificial vessel or by taking a piece of blood vessel from elsewhere in the patient's body.

With proper medical treatment, most patients who have suffered traumatic aneurysms from acupuncture accidents recover with no lasting effects.

Prevention of traumatic aneurysm

This injury can be prevented by looking and feeling for arteries before inserting needles. When you see that a blood vessel is near the desired acupoint, press the end of the thumb of your other hand into the patient's skin, gently pushing away and protecting the vessel. The thumbnail becomes a shield, as well as a guide for the needle as it is inserted.

When working over and around the deeper vessels, you must be familiar with the path of these structures. While planning a particular person's treatment, you may find it useful to refer to your anatomy books or charts, especially if you have not given acupuncture in the specific area for some time.

Watch insertion depths when working around sensitive areas such as arteries. After withdrawing needles, press these points with a cotton ball for at least 30 to 60 seconds. Take note of any bumps that have arisen after a first treatment. Also record their size and location. If, at the next treatment, a bump has disappeared, it means a small haematoma has been reabsorbed. If it has grown or is causing discomfort, consider the possibility that a blood vessel was pierced during the previous treatment.

If a patient has a history of any coagulation disorder, you will want to choose fewer points and reduce the depth of needle insertion.

Advise patients with a bit of bleeding under the skin to place an ice pack over the area to stop bleeding. You may also prescribe herbs that stop bleeding, such as Yunnan White Medicine. If the mass continues to grow, indicating damage to a larger vessel or arterial branch, send the patient to a physician or emergency immediately.

ARTERIOVENOUS FISTULA

Case study 1.19

A 38-year-old woman suffering from neck pain and headaches accepted a neighbour's offer to use a sewing needle to pierce the LI-4 point on the left hand. This do-it-yourself acupuncture treatment was deep and resulted in considerable bleeding. The following day, there was a large bruise on the 'patient's' hand. The bruise went away, but a month later a varicose vein developed in the area. The woman's middle and ring finger were purplish, and the fine motor skills of that hand deteriorated. At hospital, an arteriovenous fistula was diagnosed and surgery was performed to repair the wound (Shao 1977).

Related acupoints

Refer to Table 1.1.

Discussion of arteriovenous fistula

An arteriovenous fistula is an abnormal channel between an artery and a vein. It may be congenital, but is more commonly caused by any injury that damages an artery and a vein that lie next to each other. The injury is typically a piercing wound, such as stabbing with a knife, but in rare cases an acupuncture needle has punctured both an artery and a vein, forming a passage between the two.

Although this case involves LI-4, in theory a fistula could come up anywhere on the body where a needle can be driven into an artery and a vein. At LI-4, for example, there is a dorsal venous network (the beginning of the cephalic vein) and the radial artery's palmar branch. Because the arterial pressure is higher, blood is forced into the vein and the surrounding tissues. The vein walls bulge. Swelling and bruising can come up quite quickly, or take days to develop.

What to do in case of arteriovenous fistula

In all cases, this is a situation that requires surgical repair. After surgery, physiotherapy and exercise are needed to restore full function to the affected area.

Prevention of arteriovenous fistula

Awareness of the anatomy of blood vessels in the treatment area is a key to prevention. The acupuncturist can avoid puncturing vessels by making sure the needle is not inserted too far. A sensation of elastic resistance to the needle is a warning sign for the practitioner; the patient may also complain of a sharp pain. It is bad enough to puncture one vessel. Hitting a vein and an artery in one stroke can have more serious repercussions. Withdraw the needle and firmly press on the point for a minimum of 2 minutes with a sterile cotton ball. A pressure dressing applied for a couple of hours will generally prevent the wound from forming a channel for blood flow and keep a fistula from forming. If you have any reason to suspect this is occurring anyway, your follow-up with the patient may also include a suggestion that the wound be checked by a physician.

ORBITAL BRUISING ('PANDA BEAR EYES')

There are many acupoints around the eyes (Fig. 1.13), and a large number of these are in daily use. Recent reports indicate that acupuncture is effective to various degrees in treating such eye conditions as macular degeneration, eyelid spasm, dry eyes, deterioration of vision and changes related to aging. If there is an injury to this area, the special character of the tissues causes bleeding to develop quickly; the subsequent bruise, which may cover half or even the whole orbital circle, suggests the common Chinese name for this injury.

Case study 1.20

Most practising acupuncturists will eventually give a patient a case of 'panda bear eyes'. Its effects are cosmetic and temporary, so we don't find it written up in journals. I recorded this particular case in my work notes after it came up in a discussion with a colleague.

It concerns an acupuncturist who treated a patient's headaches by needling, among other points, Ex. Tai Yang. There was a tiny amount of bleeding – a common occurrence in such a case – when the needle was withdrawn. The practitioner pressed the spot with a sterile cotton ball, and sent the patient home with a suggestion to apply compresses several times over the next couple of days. A few hours after the treatment, the subcutaneous bleeding spread a large and ugly-looking bruise over the patient's temple and around one eye. The aggrieved patient had a photograph taken, and in due course the acupuncturist was summoned to court to explain his actions. The patient was awarded compensation. Although orbital bruising presents no significant danger to the patient's health, it is worth discussing how to prevent and handle this situation simply because it occurs with such frequency in the normal course of practice.

Figure 1.13 Acupoints around the eye.

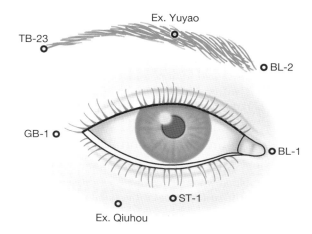

Related acupoints

ST-1, ST-2
BL-1, BL-2
TB-23
GB-1
Ex. Yu Yao, Ex. Qiu Hou and Ex. Tai Yang

Discussion of orbital bruising

The eye area is richly supplied with blood, as it is surrounded by a fine network of shallow blood vessels. Be aware of orbital vasculature. Beneath ST-2, there are branches of the facial artery and vein, and the infraorbital artery and vein.

Beneath BL-1 lie the supraorbital artery, which comes from the ophthalmic artery, the angular artery from the facial artery, and accompanying veins. Under BL-2 are the supraorbital artery and vein. The superficial branches of the temporal artery and vein lie beneath TB-23. Ex. Yu Yao is in the vicinity of the frontal artery and vein, and Ex. Qiu Hou is near the infraorbital artery and vein.

The orbits are bony cavities containing the eyeballs, muscles, nerves, blood vessels, fat and structures that produce and drain tears. The eyeball is cushioned by soft subcutaneous tissue that is quite loose and contains many tiny blood vessels, so even when needling is shallow it can easily cause bleeding. There is nowhere for the blood to go, except toward the surface. Because the tissue around the eye is so pliable, and because there are no big strong muscles there to contract and stop the bleeding, the blood spreads out easily over a large area. This results in impressive 'shiners'. Bleeding is of course worse in people who are taking aspirin or anticoagulants.

The patient is also likely to experience discomfort from the swelling of the tissues themselves, and because the pressure of blood in the orbital cavity makes the eyeball feel as though it is bulging out. The swelling often restricts the movement of the eyelid. These symptoms are upsetting to the patient, who may feel the acupuncturist has caused an injury and something should be done about it. Although a black eye often looks far worse than it is, we need to be sensitive to the fact that, for some people, even such a temporary, cosmetic injury adversely affects them socially or professionally.

What to do in case of orbital bruising

If a small artery or vein around the eye is perforated, there may be some drops of blood when the needle is withdrawn, or a small swelling or lump may come up. The surface area of the skin looks normal, and the patient will not feel any discomfort or subjective symptoms. But a couple of hours later a bruise will begin to develop and spread. As the panda bear eyes become more and more noticeable to others, the patient becomes a walking billboard, advertising the fact that he or she has just had acupuncture.

If there is more subcutaneous bleeding, the eyelid will feel swollen, and the patient will have trouble opening and closing the eye. Sometimes when the needle breaks a slightly deeper vessel, especially when we work on Ex. Qiu Hou, the bony eye socket restricts the space where the blood can flow, so the pressure of blood pooling behind and around the eye pushes the eyeball outward, causing an uncomfortable 'bug-eyed' sensation. As circulation is impeded, the patient may also have blurred vision.

It takes 2 to 3 weeks for the bruise to be absorbed and the swelling to disappear. Vision and eye movement will return to normal.

If you see bruising or the patient calls in later to report it, the proper treatment is a cold eye compress placed on the affected area for 20 minutes, three times a day. The patient should be advised to avoid heavy athletic activity, housework or other physical exertion for a couple of days, because that may aggravate the bleeding. If the bruise is small, after 24 hours the cold compresses should be replaced by warm ones, twice a day for 20 minutes each time. For a large bruise, it is preferable to wait for 36 hours before applying heat. The warmth will encourage the body to reabsorb the blood. Gentle massage around the orbit will also promote circulation. If the patient is experiencing vision problems, we may suggest that an eye patch is worn for a few days to protect the eye from harsh light. Artificial tears can also be used to keep the eye moist.

If the patient's eye is bulging uncomfortably, suggest a consultation with a physician or eye specialist, who may apply a pressure bandage and prescribe other therapies to stop the bleeding. Normally, extreme bulging happens only in a person who has a blood coagulation disease such as haemophilia. The application of pressure over the eye can cause damage if done incorrectly, so it should only be performed by a trained medical professional. It is unwise for an acupuncturist to attempt this.

Prevention of orbital bruising

A thin needle, shallow insertion and gentle stimulation are the primary factors in preventing bleeding around the eye. When treating any of the points listed above, it is recommended to use gauge 36 (0.20 mm diameter, 13 mm long) needles. If the angle will be oblique, insert the needle up to half of its length, in other words about 6 mm. If the angle of insertion is flatter relative to the skin, a safe depth is up to two-thirds of the needle's length – approximately 8 mm. Stimulation should be very gentle, and in a tiny range of movement.

Needles should be retained in these points for a shorter length of time than for points on the rest of the body. For points such as BL-1, GB-1, ST-1 and Ex. Qiu Hou, which are located in very loose tissue that is rich in blood vessels, it is suggested that needles should be left in for only 5 to 10 minutes. Needles can be retained in BL-2, ST-2, TB-23, Ex. Yu Yao and Ex. Tai Yang for 10 to 15 minutes. A needle in any acupoint sets off a reflex effect in vessels and nerves, which results in flushing and congestion of the skin and subcutaneous tissue. The longer the needles are in, especially in an area that is richly supplied with tiny vessels, the more flushing occurs. This increases the likelihood of bleeding.

For sensitive points around the eyes, practitioners should use a special incremental withdrawal technique. This means partially withdrawing the needle and allowing it to stay there for a minute or so while occupying ourselves with something else. Continue to withdraw the needle in small stages – as many as three for very sensitive points – to allow the tiny vessels to close up behind it. This technique greatly reduces the risk of orbital bleeding.

After needles are removed from these points, a sterile cotton ball should be used to press on each hole for a minute or so, regardless of whether the treatment has been for tonification or reduction.

GENERAL PREVENTION AND MANAGEMENT OF BRUISING

Orbital bruising is just one example of this extremely common and generally minor occurrence in acupuncture. Besides the area around the eyes, bruises are most likely to turn up on the shoulder, elbow, wrist, upper and lower abdomen, the entire back, hip and outside of the thigh.

If you know a treatment is likely to cause bruising, especially to a patient who is particularly nervous or likely to be upset, it is advisable to warn the person in advance, and offer reassurance that the condition is temporary and does not indicate any serious damage.

To help prevent bruising, press on sensitive points longer than usual after removing the needle, regardless of whether you have done tonification or reduction techniques. If a bruise or small lump comes up anyway, first aid measures are the same as those for orbital bruising. If the bruise is more like a large lump, consider whether the patient might have haemophilia. The patient should be referred immediately to a physician.

The collection of a detailed history before treating a new patient will reveal whether the person has a history of abnormal bleeding or liver disease, or is taking blood-thinning medications, all of which increase the likelihood of bleeding under the skin.

References

Chen Yuzhen et al 1985 One case report of subarachnoid hemorrhage caused by acupuncture on neck points. Shanxi TCM Journal 1:47

Cheng Zhifang et al 1963 Jiangsu TCM Journal 10:27

Gao Xinzhu et al 1993 Acupuncture accident and its prevention. Hunan Science & Technology Publishing House, Changsha

Ilhan A, Alioglu Z, Adanir M et al 1995 Transverse myelopathy after acupuncture therapy: a case report. Acupuncture and Electro-Therapeutics Research International Journal 20:191-194

Jiang Zuoxian 1988 Adverse effects of acupuncture – 100 case studies. Shanxi TCM College Learned Journal 11(1):25

Kao Chiunglin, Chang Jenping 2002 Pseudoaneurysm of the popliteal artery: a rare sequela of acupuncture. Texas Heart Institute Journal 29(2):126-129

Liu Xinji 1981 Four cases of acupuncture accident in treatment of patients with schizophrenia. Journal of Neuropsychosis (China) (5):317

Lun Xin, Rong Li 1997 Analysing selected cases of acupuncture accidents. People's Health Publishing House, Beijing

Murata K, Nishio A, Nishikawa M, Ohinata Y, Sakaguchi M, Nishimura S 1990 Subarachnoid hemorrhage and spinal root injury caused by acupuncture needle – case report. Neurologia Medico-Chirurfica (Tokyo) 30(12):956-959

Peuker E, Gronemeyer D 2001 Rare but serious complications of acupuncture: traumatic lesions. Acupuncture in Medicine 19(2):103-108

Rampes H, James R 1995 Complications of acupuncture. Acup Med 13: 26-33

Shao Jianbin 1977 Acupuncture injury to blood vessels. Tianjin Medical Journal 12:613

Shen Zhuobin. 1983 Acupuncture experiment record. Shanxi Science & Technology Publishing House, Taiyuan.

Wang Li 1991 Hand muscle contraction following needling of PC 6: two case reports Shanghai Acupuncture Journal (2):45

Xia Chen 1993 Abnormal reaction following Chinese herb injection on acupuncture points Clinical Acupuncture Journal 2(3):75 Beijing

Zhu Ji 1990 Case of death from aorta injury, caused by acupuncture needling of LIV-14. Shanghai Acupuncture Journal 2:31

Organs

2

The most common sites of organ punctures from acupuncture are the heart, lung, liver, kidney, gall bladder and bladder.

PNEUMOTHORAX AND HAEMOPNEUMOTHORAX

The most frequently reported severe traumatic accidents caused by acupuncture needles are pneumothorax, spinal cord injuries and hepatitis (Peuker & Gronemeyer 2001, Rotchford 2004). Of these, pneumothorax is the most common. White & Ernst cite a survey of 1100 Australian practitioners of TCM, which revealed that of a total of 3222 adverse events of acupuncture in their practices – most of which were minor – there were 64 cases of pneumothorax (White & Ernst 2001).

Though none of the cases reported in the Australian survey was fatal, people can die from pneumothorax (Brettel 1981). Dr Zhou Jianwei, of Chengdu University of TCM, collected 110 cases of pneumothorax reported between 1950 and 1994, of which five resulted in death – an incidence of 4.5% (Zhou 1995).

As Rotchford points out, the literature suggests acupuncture-related pneumothorax is rare or is only associated with incompetence. In my opinion, the number of cases is still significant enough to deserve detailed examination here.

Case study 2.1

In one case, a 31-year-old pregnant woman sought acupuncture treatment for asthma. The acupoints chosen were on her back, and as the needles were inserted she experienced severe pains in the lung region. Shortly after the treatment, the woman began to have difficulty in breathing, and her rate of respiration increased. She was admitted to hospital in severe respiratory distress, resulting from pneumothorax of both lungs. She recovered after treatment (Wright et al 1991).

Case study 2.2

A 26-year-old female complaining of pain in her right shoulder went for acupuncture. The acupuncturist chose, among other points, SI-13 for treatment. After the points had been marked, but before the needling, the patient moved her arm (Fig. 2.1). Therefore the sites marked on the skin no longer lined up with the proper acupoints. Because the scapula had been moved by the change in arm position, the lung was punctured by needling of SI-13.

Three hours after the treatment, the patient began feeling chest pressure and shortness of breath, as well as pain in the right side of the chest, which radiated to the upper back and which was aggravated by coughing. The woman went to hospital, and the attending physician found diminished respiratory sounds from the right lung, and that her trachea had shifted to the left. An X-ray showed the right lung had collapsed 30%, a clear picture of pneumothorax.

Treatment consisted of abstraction of 500 ml of air from the right pleural cavity, and a course of antibiotics and cough suppressant. Before her discharge from hospital a week later, an X-ray showed the patient's lung had returned to normal (Bairen 1987).

Case study 2.3

Another case of pneumothorax cited in reviews of adverse reactions after acupuncture involves a 29-year-old woman with back pain. Ten minutes after acupuncture treatment, she experienced breathing difficulties, and severe pain that radiated from the acupoint on her back to the front of the chest wall. The review doesn't specify which point, but it was likely one of the back shu points on the Bladder meridian. An X-ray revealed a 30–40% pneumothorax, which was successfully treated by the insertion of chest tubes (Mazal et al 1980).

Related acupoints

LU-1, LU-2
ST-11, ST-12, ST-13, ST-14, ST-15, ST-16, ST-18, ST-19
SP-17, SP-18, SP-19, SP-20, SP-21
SI-12, SI-13, SI-14, SI-15
BL-11 to BL-21, BL-41 to BL-50,
KI-22, KI-23, KI-24, KI-25, KI-26, KI-27
PC-1
GB-21, GB-22, GB-23, GB-24, GB-25
LIV-13, LIV-14
LI-16, LI-17
TB-15
Ren-15, Ren-22
Ex. Jing Bi or Bi Cong, Ex. Ding Chuan, Ex.Yi Shu or Wei Guan Xia Shu

Discussion of pneumothorax

It is a common misconception that the lungs are safely protected behind the clavicle and within the ribcage. In fact, the inner top corners of the lungs extend 2 to 3 cm above the clavicle, where they are close to the surface of the body (Figs 2.2, 2.3). They also lie close to the surface from the sixth intercostal

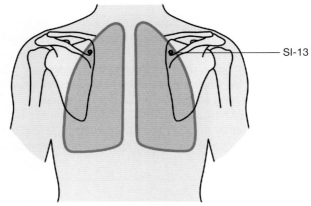

Posterior

Figure 2.1a Take care the patient's position for point location remains unchanged when needling. When the patient's arm is down, there is no danger from needling SI-13 because the lung is protected by the scapula bone.

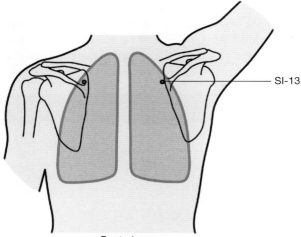

Posterior

Figure 2.1b If the patient's arm is lifted, the scapula moves laterally, and a needle in SI-13 can puncture the pleura and cause pneumothorax.

space at the midclavicular line on inspiration, to the eighth intercostal space at the midaxillary line, and to the 11th intercostal space at the back during quiet respiration. Their posterior border runs along a line from where the scapular line meets the 10th rib, down to the 10th thoracic vertebra.

Whereas the upper part of the pleural cavity fits snugly against the lungs, its bottom section hangs lower than the lungs, by about the width of two ribs. Care must be taken to avoid lung puncture when needling points in all of these areas.

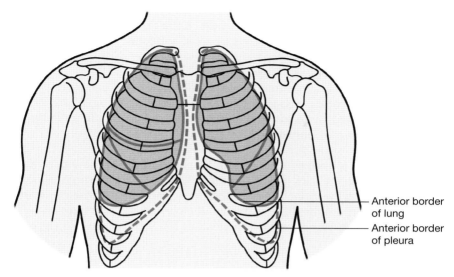

Figure 2.2 Anterior surface projection of the lungs.

The practitioner must also be careful when treating patients with emphysema, asthma or chronic bronchitis, because the lung and pleural cavity are likely to be enlarged as a result of these diseases. This increases the risk of puncture.

Pneumothorax is a pocket of air between the two layers of pleura. Incorrect needling of any of the related points can cause pneumothorax or haemo-pneumothorax (if blood vessels are damaged). In theory, pneumothorax can be

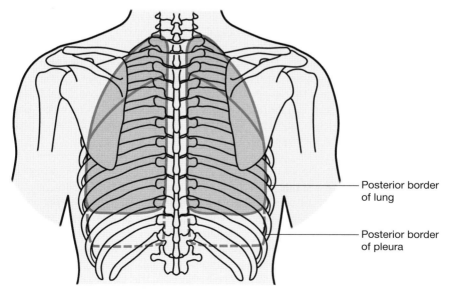

Figure 2.3 Posterior surface projection of the lungs.

caused by puncturing the parietal pleura – the outside layer – or the visceral pleura, which is the layer that lies next to the lung. When air is introduced between these two layers, it forms a pocket, and exerts pressure that can collapse the lung.

If death occurs, it is from airway blockage by blood and mucus. Usually, either the tracheal cartilage or the lung through the visceral pleura has been punctured. Blood leaks into the trachea or air rushes into the pleural cavity's negative space, collapsing the lung.

How can something as thin as an acupuncture needle cause pneumothorax? After all, the thick, elastic chest muscle would close off such a minuscule wound instantly. In fact, the air does not come from outside the body. In acupuncture, if a needle goes through the pleurae and punctures one of the alveoli, air will be sucked *from* the lung by the vacuum between the pleural layers.

As the apex of the lung extends higher than the clavicle, it is very easy to wound the top of the lung if the depth and angle of penetration are not correct when treating points just above the clavicle on either side of the trachea, such as GB-21, LI-16, LI-17 and TB-15.

When a person takes a breath, the expansion and contraction of the lungs are quite large movements. On a deep inhalation, the lower border of the lung can descend as much as the width of a rib. So if we needle BL-20, BL-21, BL-49 or BL-50 there is danger of puncturing the lung if the depth and angle of penetration are not correct. Also, when needling points between the scapula and the spine, if the patient moves his or her arm, the scapula will move laterally, exposing an area between the edge of the bone and the spine through which the lung can be reached. SI-12 and SI-13 are the risky points in this case.

When treating points on the back, side or front of the chest, ask the patient to avoid changing position or taking deep breaths. Also, during the time when the needle is retained in these points, if the patient has an uncontrollable urge to cough or sneeze, the practitioner needs to observe carefully, and either back off the needle's depth or even remove needles from the more sensitive areas to avoid causing a pneumothorax.

A pneumothorax may develop during a treatment or shortly thereafter. Symptoms include a sudden, sharp chest or back pain, a sudden dry, hacking cough and shortness of breath. If, after acupuncture, the patient complains of shoulder pain on the same side that was treated, and this pain was not there before acupuncture, practitioners should be alert to the possibility that this may be the only presenting symptom of a pneumothorax. Acupuncturists must also be aware that signs of a pneumothorax may not be evident for up to 24 hours after treatment, as it takes some time for the air pocket to develop between the pleural layers. The second case cited above is an example of this.

What to do in case of pneumothorax

A small pneumothorax usually does not require treatment. In most cases, the lung shrinks by less than 20% and the air is reabsorbed within a few days without intervention. In cases where more than 20% of the lung has collapsed, the patient needs to have the air suctioned out at the hospital, any fluids drained and antibiotics administered. A patient with a suspected pneumothorax with few or mild symptoms can be sent home to rest, with regular monitoring by the practitioner. However, if symptoms worsen over the course of 10–12 hours from their initial appearance, the patient should be sent to a physician or hospital emergency department for an X-ray.

Prevention of pneumothorax

Most cases of acupuncture-related pneumothorax could be prevented if the practitioner had had a better knowledge of anatomy. Always bear in mind where the borders of the pleurae and the lungs are situated, and the thickness of the soft tissue covering them. Before placing needles in these sensitive areas, check the depth and angle of insertion, and train yourself to become familiar with the 'feel' of different tissues touched by the needle. For example, when the needle touches the trachea under Ren-22, there will be a sense of elastic resistance, the patient may feel a tickle deep in the throat and have a desire to cough. If a needle touches a pulsing artery, you may be able to feel this movement. Withdraw the needle from these structures to avoid injuring the patient.

Electrical stimulation of these related points requires even more caution. Even when the angle and depth of the needle are correct, the weight of the electrical connector may subtly change the needle's direction. The pulses from the stimulator can also cause the needle to vibrate, which may change its position.

Be aware of which patients may be at greater risk for pneumothorax. These include smokers, people who are tall and slim, particularly males, patients with emphysema, patients who are or have been taking corticosteroids, patients with active cancer and anyone who has an abnormally small amount of body fat, for any reason.

About spontaneous pneumothorax

It is possible for a simple pneumothorax to occur spontaneously, when a part of a lung has been weakened by diving or high-altitude flying. People with pre-existing health problems, especially lung diseases such as those mentioned above, may develop a more serious but still spontaneous pneumothorax; the fact that it develops after acupuncture may simply be a coincidence. However, to be on the safe side with patients who are at greater risk, I substitute the following points for those on the back and the chest: LU-5, LU-7, LU-9, ST-36, KI-3, etc.

That way, if the patient develops a cough, chest pain or shortness of breath after acupuncture, I can be confident this situation has arisen spontaneously or is related to a cold or flu, and is not the result of an acupuncture accident.

In his review, Dr Rotchford (2004) concludes that one can see how easily a case of spontaneous pneumothorax could be blamed inaccurately on acupuncture. The odds of a spontaneous occurrence may be as high as what some literature reports as being associated with acupuncture. This would be especially true in a high-risk group such as tall male smokers.

However, Rotchford also points out that pneumothorax may be easily missed – and therefore underreported – by health practitioners who are not aware that shoulder pain may be the only presenting symptom.

HEART INJURY

An injury to the heart is of course one of the most serious accidents that can occur. Although these are quite rare, when they do occur, they are often fatal. Of four cases reviewed by Dr Zhou in China, all had died. Peuker & Gronemeyer (2001) cite eight cases of heart injury from acupuncture accidents written up in the scientific literature between 1965 and 2001; two of these patients died.

Heart injuries generally involve a puncture to a major cardiac blood vessel, or to the wall of the heart itself. These injuries then result in bleeding, causing shock, myocardial ischaemia, cardiac tamponade and heart failure. If the structure of the heart itself is damaged, functional problems such as arrhythmia, a reduction of cardiac output and pulmonary oedema will result. Considering the serious consequences of an accidental heart puncture, acupuncturists must treat related points with great caution, as we see in the following cases.

Case study 2.4

An 83-year-old emaciated female with no prior history of heart disease was given acupuncture, with a 3 cun needle inserted into the middle third of the sternum. Twenty minutes after treatment, the patient's heart rate slowed down and she lost consciousness. In hospital, echocardiography revealed cardiac tamponade with collapse of the right atrium and ventricle. Surgery was needed to stop the oozing of blood from a lesion in the anterior wall of the ventricle. The woman recovered and was discharged after 2 weeks (Kirchgatterer et al 2000).

Case study 2.5

The patient was a 19-year-old woman admitted to hospital for treatment of schizophrenia. Acupuncture was given once a day for 10 days, employing among others the points Ren-15 and LI-11. On the eighth treatment, as usual, the practitioner used a 2 cun needle to work on Ren-15, inserting it perpendicular to the skin; once through the skin the needle was pushed 1 cm at an upward angle toward the sternum. Electrical stimulation was connected to these two points. The practitioner observed the needle in Ren-15 was moving – a sign that it was in contact with the heart muscle. After several minutes, the patient screamed, her head arched back, and she vomited. The needle was immediately removed. Cyanosis was evident on her face, and her heart and respiration stopped.

Open cardiac massage was used to restart breathing and heartbeat, but the patient remained in a coma until she died from a heart rupture and lung infection 20 days later. A review of this case concluded the needle in Ren-15 punctured the patient's heart (Liu Xinji 1981).

Case study 2.6

Another fatal case involved a 40-year-old woman who was being treated for fibromyalgia. An experienced practitioner inserted a needle into her sternum at the level of the fourth intercostal space. A few minutes later, the patient complained of chest pain and she was rushed to hospital, where efforts to resuscitate her were unsuccessful. A postmortem found blood in the pericardial cavity, and a perforation in the anterior wall of the right ventricle. An X-ray of the woman's chest showed a sternal foramen just at the level of the acupoint. This phenomenon will be discussed in more detail later in this section. (Halvorsen et al 1995).

Related acupoints

ST-15, ST-16, ST-17, ST-18, ST-19, ST-20, ST-21
SP-17, SP-18, SP-19, SP-20
KI-21, KI-22, KI-23, KI-24, KI-25
PC-1
LIV-14
Ren-14, Ren-15, Ren-16 (only if a patient has a congenital sternal foramen)
    (Some points in this list are dangerous only if the patient has a disease that enlarges the heart. Others are only risky if the needle is placed at an incorrect angle. See discussion section for more detail on this issue.)

Discussion of heart injury

The heart is situated obliquely in the chest, with the attached end directed upward, backward and to the right (Fig. 2.4). The apex of the heart points downward, forward and to the left. The heart is placed behind the lower two-thirds of the sternum, and sits more to the left side of the chest cavity.

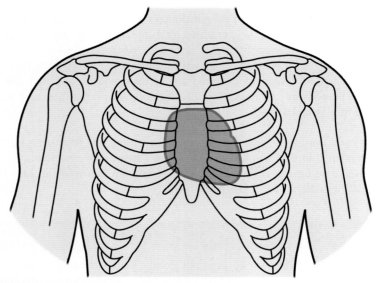

Figure 2.4 Surface projection of the heart.

For a more detailed projection, imagine the heart has four corners. Normally its surface projects to these coordinates. The left upper corner touches the inferior border of the left second costal cartilage, 1.2 cm left of the edge of the sternum. The left lower corner – the apex of the heart – is at the left fifth intercostal space, 1 to 2 cm left of the midclavicular line. The right upper corner is at the superior border of the right third costal cartilage, 1 cm from the right edge of the sternum, and the right lower corner is normally located at the right sixth sternocostal joint.

Most cases of heart injuries come from carelessness and lack of anatomical knowledge on the part of the practitioner. The two main errors are in the depth and the angle of needle insertion. The chest wall itself is not thick, so if the patient is small or thin, the distance from the skin surface to the heart is even shorter (Fig. 2.5).

'A postmortem showed that the distance from the skin to the posterior surface of the sternum was 13–19 mm.' (Rosted 2004).

The distance from the skin to the sternum, in general, is probably less than 1 cm. That is why using even a 1.5 cun needle can cause heart injury.

When we insert the needle, most of the time we use the fingers of our other hand to stretch, press and fix the skin to keep it in position for the needle. This further compresses the soft tissue, a point that the acupuncturist must take into account when gauging the proper depth, in order to reduce the risk of heart puncture.

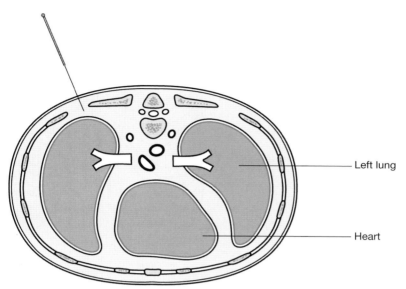

Figure 2.5 Transverse section of the thoracic cavity showing the lungs and heart. Theoretically, it is possible to injure the heart through the back, but it would take a serious degree of practitioner ignorance to do this, as the needle would have to perforate the pleural cavity and lungs first. Injury is more likely through the chest wall.

Also, when the heart itself is already diseased, resulting in enlargement or hydropericardium, this further increases the danger of injury from acupuncture.

There is risk, also, in treating patients with myocarditis or constrictive pericarditis or any other condition that results in degeneration, looseness, swelling, adhesions or calcification of the heart muscle itself. Any scar tissue or changes in the texture or strength of the heart muscle increases the risk of injury.

Some practitioners, when treating patients with chronic pain, like to use a technique of embedding needles in acupoints on the neck, back or chest. These may be special needles that look like a thumbtack, or may be ordinary acupuncture needles whose handles have been cut off. These are fixed in place with a piece of adhesive for a considerable period of time. The danger is that these needles may be forgotten and left in for far longer than is acceptable, and can eventually travel to organs such as the heart. Several cases of embedded or semipermanent needles working their way into the heart are reported in the literature (Kataota 1997).

Another potential hazard of which acupuncturists should become aware is the possibility that a patient has a congenital sternal foramen, as in the third case cited above (Fig. 2.6). The foramen is a congenital abnormality due to an incomplete fusion of the sternal plates.

Figure 2.6 Congenital sternal foramen.

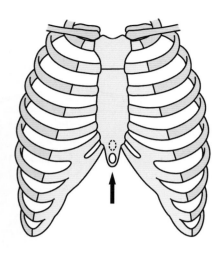

According to Peuker & Gronemeyer (2001), it exists in 5–8% of the population. Other studies suggest as much as 9.6% of men and 4.3% of women have this condition (McCormick 1981). The foramen is usually located at the level of the fourth intercostal space (precisely at the acupoint Ren-17). A standard X-ray may not show it (Peuker & Gronemeyer 2001). The needle could easily pass through the connective tissue of the foramen and puncture the heart, causing cardiac tamponade.

Symptoms of heart injury are: severe chest pain, difficulty breathing, paleness, cyanosis in the lips, fainting, shock and convulsions. Blood pressure may drop suddenly, and respiration may cease. If puncture results in a cardiac tamponade, the patient may exhibit shortness of breath, dysphoria and a weak pulse; an X-ray may indicate enlargement of the heart. In addition, the patient may have symptoms of functional insufficiency, such as arrhythmia, chest distress and a cough that produces blood. The end result, if not treated immediately, will be heart failure.

What to do in case of heart injury

Heart punctures from acupuncture have resulted in death, in several reported cases. If a patient becomes pale, complains of chest pain and difficulty in breathing, and you see a needle rhythmically moving, stop treatment immediately, press on the point, closely watch your patient and call an ambulance.

As a practitioner, you must be alert to the signs of a heart injury, and if these symptoms occur it is your responsibility to call for medical assistance immediately so that the patient can be treated as soon as possible. Delayed treatment could be fatal. As we saw in the first case above, even when the patient requires surgery to repair the damage, successful recuperation is possible if treatment is begun promptly.

Prevention of heart injury

Questioning new patients about their medical history, especially of heart and lung problems, is imperative in prevention of serious injuries. If you suspect, or the patient reports, a heart condition you can percuss the chest to hear the heart's actual size. Many diseases, such as cardiomegaly, cardiac effusion and myocarditis, can cause the heart to enlarge. Some people are born with abnormal hearts.

Most people will not know if they have a sternal foramen, and it is not easy for the practitioner to detect. If a needle being inserted into the sternal area goes in more deeply than common sense would dictate, given that there is supposed to be a bone there, it is wise to suspect a foramen. It is a good idea, when treating areas around the heart, to use shorter needles – 0.5–1 cun – just to be on the safe side.

When we treat chest points that are located in the intercostal space, it is important to insert the needles at a slightly oblique angle, rather than perpendicular to the body surface. If the patient is less muscled or thinner, this angle should be even more horizontal, relative to the skin.

Always insert the needles in the direction toward the outside of the body, rather than toward the midline. Ensure that no more than 1 cm of the needle is penetrating under the skin.

When needling Ren-14 or Ren-15, the direction of insertion should be slightly oblique, and toward the navel, rather than toward the heart.

When treating back points, for instance on the Bladder meridian, the needle should be inserted obliquely either into the large muscle structures on either side of the spine (such as Ex. Hua Tuo Jia Ji points, which are needled into the muscles) or toward the outside of the body.

Always proceed slowly and gently when inserting the needle; observe the patient's reaction carefully and ask for feedback, especially when the person is lying face down. Do not try to force the needle to get the sensation of de qi. Wait for it to arrive. Some cases of injury have resulted from the practitioner vigorously stimulating and moving the needle to connect with de qi.

LIVER INJURY

The liver is soft and solid, but its surface is friable and easily lacerated. It is full of blood and bile. Therefore, if it is punctured with a needle, blood and bile will leak into the abdominal cavity, resulting in peritonitis. If this is not treated promptly, it is life threatening.

It should be pointed out that in normal circumstances most of the adult liver is shielded by the costal arch, except for the section under the xiphoid

Case study 2.7

A female, aged 40, came for acupuncture to relieve stomach aches after meals. The practitioner put needles into Ren-12, Ren-13 and Ren-15. During the whole treatment, the patient complained of feeling sharp internal pain under these three points. The acupuncturist removed the needles, which relieved the woman's discomfort. She went home and slept. In the middle of the night, the woman was awakened by pain in the upper abdomen, and went to hospital 12 hours after the acupuncture treatment. In addition to the pain, she had difficulty in breathing, nausea, thirst and restlessness. The examining physician observed facial pallor and distension of the abdomen. The stomach muscles were tight, with rebound tenderness. Fluid was extracted from the patient's abdominal cavity to check for the presence of bile and blood. Blood was found, and exploratory surgery was performed. It was found that the left lobe of the liver, directly under the above-mentioned acupoints, had been wounded and was bleeding. After a left lobectomy and further treatment during 50 days in hospital, the patient recovered (Feng 1965).

Related acupoints

When the following points are needled, the liver can be injured even if it is healthy:

Ren-14, Ren-15
ST-18, ST-19
GB-24
LIV-14.

When the liver is diseased it can be enlarged, which increases the danger of injury when needling these points:

Ren-11, Ren-12, Ren-13
ST-20, ST-21, ST-22, ST-23, ST-24, ST-25
GB-25, GB-26
LIV-13
SP-15, SP-16, SP-17, SP-21
KI-20, KI-21, KI-22.

process. Different diseases can cause the organ to enlarge, making it even more vulnerable to puncture where it is not protected by the ribs.

Discussion of liver injury

The liver is the largest gland in the body, and is located in the upper right part of the abdominal cavity. In a normal liver, the upper border runs from the seventh intercostal space on the right midaxillary line to the fifth intercostal space on the midclavicular line, to the xiphosternal joint on the midline, to the fifth costal cartilage on the left midclavicular line (Fig. 2.7).

The lower border runs from the 11th intercostal space on the right mid-axillary line along the lower border of the costal arch to the costocartilage joint of the eighth and ninth ribs, to 3 cm directly below the xiphoid process, and on an oblique line up to the left, meeting the upper border at the fifth costal cartilage.

The surface projection of the liver varies according to different people's body shape and build. In a short and overweight person, the transverse diameter of the liver will be longer; the left corner of the organ can reach to the left midclavicle line and the entire organ lies higher in the body, so its lower edge may be even with the lower margin of the costal arch, which makes it difficult for the practitioner to feel where it is.

A tall, thin person, on the other hand, has a liver whose transverse diameter is very short. Its left corner may reach only as far as the body midline, or even less. And the liver's lower edge can drop down, where it is easy for the practitioner to locate and feel. This means that when your patient is tall and slender, the fact that the liver is more exposed and the person's muscle layer is thinner makes it easier to puncture the organ if you are not very careful about needle placement. When a tall, slim person comes through the clinic door, the experienced practitioner is immediately aware that extra care must be taken in accurately locating and needling near organs.

It is very difficult to injure the liver from needling acupuncture points in the back, because the left longitudinal sulcus, connective tissues such as ligaments

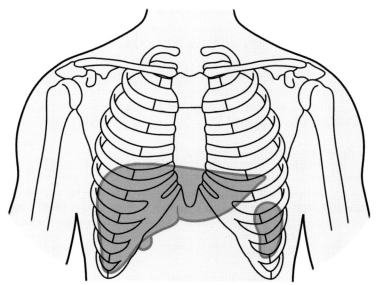

Figure 2.7 Surface projection of the liver (also including the gall bladder and spleen).

and the oesophagus lie between the back wall and the liver. Therefore, the risk comes mainly from points on the side of the body and the abdomen.

Normally, in an adult, the liver is palpable only 3 to 5 cm under the xiphoid process, the rest being covered by the costal arch. However, different diseases can cause the organ to enlarge. If we can feel the liver below the costal arch, it indicates some pathological swelling. In children, the liver is normally lower, so it is palpable below the costal arch.

The liver can actually move in a range of 2–3 cm, downward when the person is standing or inhaling, and upward when he or she is lying down or exhaling.

When the liver is swollen, the surface area in contact with the body surface is considerably larger than normal. This means that the danger of puncture is higher, and the number of acupuncture points that present a risk is greater. When the liver is enlarged, its top border can reach as high as the fourth and fifth inter-costal space – the level of the diaphragm. Its lower border can extend to the umbilicus. Acupoints that are perfectly safe on a normal healthy person can become chancy when treating a patient with an enlarged liver.

Also, liver tissues whose texture has changed because of degeneration or cirrhosis are more vulnerable to injury. A liver hardened by cirrhosis can be ruptured if punctured by a needle.

Technique is important as well. Incorrect depth and direction on insertion of the needle, or repeated, aggressive lifting, thrusting or rotation after inser-tion can damage the liver. The case shown above is an example of what can occur when a needle is placed too deeply or manipulated too roughly. Since the liver is full of blood, the many liver injuries reported caused bleeding, resulting in haemorrhagic peritonitis. Signs of peritoneal irritation are stom-ach pain, abdominal wall resistance and rebound tenderness.

If, after acupuncture treatment on any of the vulnerable points, the patient experiences pain in the stomach, rigid abdominal muscles, rebound tenderness, facial pallor, nausea and vomiting, thirst, restlessness or shock, it is likely the liver has been punctured.

What to do in case of liver injury

If you suspect a liver injury, remove the needle, ask the patient to lie still, and send the patient to a physician or emergency ward. The doctors may do an X-ray, abdominal paracentesis or ultrasound examination. There may be bleed-ing that needs to be stopped, or the patient may require antibiotics.

Prevention of liver injury

If you have any suspicion your patient has a history of liver disease (including drug or alcohol abuse, or having lived or travelled where hepatitis risk is high) it is advisable to take a detailed history, and to palpate the liver to check its size and position before treating any of the points listed above. If you believe your patient has cirrhosis or any enlargement of the liver, choose your treatment points with caution, avoiding those that may touch the projecting regions of the organ. There are points on the legs and arms that will serve the same treatment functions without the risk.

Prevent liver injury with careful needling regarding angle and depth. Focus carefully on the sensation of your fingers as you insert the needles to ensure the needles are penetrating only as far as the fatty and muscle tissues, and stop before you feel an empty space sensation.

Also, it is advisable to remove clothing over the patient's abdominal area so that you get a good view of the needle and can observe its direction, depth and any movement. It is best to put the patient in a supine position when points around the liver are being treated, so the abdominal muscles stay relaxed. This will avoid having the needle inadvertently change direction through muscle movement. Ask the patient to remain still, and to tell you if he or she needs to change position, so you can assist the movement and maintain careful observation of the needles.

When working on liver area points, always insert the needles at an oblique angle, pointing slightly downward along the line of the intercostal space, and toward the outside of the body. In very thin people, the angle of the needle relative to the body surface should be even smaller, but still pointed toward the patient's side, not toward the midline of the body.

GALL BLADDER INJURY

A review of the literature to date reveals reports of acupuncture-related injury to the gall bladder. When a perforation of the gall bladder occurs, bile leaks into the peritoneal cavity and leads to biliary peritonitis. This has serious consequences. In all of the eight cases of punctured gall bladder reported in Chinese literature from 1950 to the end of the 1980s, exploratory laparotomy was performed, and either cholecystectomy or cholecystostomy was needed. All the patients recovered, but biliary peritonitis is life threatening if not treated promptly.

Case study 2.8

A male, aged 60, sought treatment to relieve acid reflux and pain in the right upper stomach. The acupuncturist worked on LIV-14, GB-24 and ST-19. Immediately after treatment, the patient's pain worsened, and several hours later it had spread to the entire abdomen.

The following day, the patient went to hospital, exhibiting signs of shock: blood pressure was 60/40, temperature was 38.8 C and pulse was 120. The doctor

continued overpage

continued

subsequently extracted 5 ml of yellow fluid from the abdominal cavity – evidence of bile leakage and peritonitis. The patient required a blood transfusion and intravenous antibiotics, and a laparotomy was carried out, during which an additional 200 ml of bilious fluid was extracted from the abdominal cavity. The surgeon also discovered the liver was enlarged, approximately 5 cm (2") below the right costal arch. The gall bladder was inflamed and enlarged to the size of a tennis ball, and bile was leaking from a perforation on the fundus of this organ. The wound precisely matched the level of acupoint ST-19.

Three peanut-sized gallstones and one roundworm were discovered in the common bile duct. These were evidently the cause of the liver and gall bladder inflammation and the abdominal pain that had caused the patient to seek treatment in the first place. A cholecystectomy and T-drainage of the common bile duct were performed. The patient subsequently recovered (Chen et al 1963).

Related acupoints

ST-19, ST-20
GB-24
LIV-13, LIV-14

If the gall bladder is enlarged these points have a risk of injury:

ST-21
Ren-12, Ren-13, Ren-14.

Discussion of gall bladder injury

The gall bladder is a small pear-shaped organ that stores and concentrates bile, which flows from the liver through the bile ducts, hepatic duct and cystic duct. It is tucked under the right lobe of the liver, its fundus projecting outward from the larger organ's anterior border. Its surface touches the intersection of the lateral edge of the straight muscle of the abdomen, and the right inter-costal arch immediately below the ninth costal cartilage. (See Fig. 2.7 for the surface projection of the gall bladder.)

Because the gall bladder lies deep within the body, protected by the liver, acupuncture can not normally harm it. However, the surface projection of the gall bladder's fundus is not always fixed. Depending on the elasticity of an individual's connective tissue, the fundus can in fact move up and down into a more vulnerable position. The size of the gall bladder also varies in size from one person to another. In a short and stout person, the gall bladder usually sits in a higher and more lateral position. In a thin, tall person, the organ will be lower and positioned closer to the midline. This means that when we are treating acupoints on the stomach and chest of a thin person we must take into account not only the body's fat and muscle covering, but the position of the gall bladder, which may be unusually close to the centre of the body.

Also, if the gall bladder is enlarged because of inflammation, gallstones or a tumour, or is pushed out of its usual position by an enlarged liver, it becomes more vulnerable to puncture. It is quite common, in clinical practice, to feel a gall bladder that has been shifted out of place by hepatomegaly.

The case study cited above is an example of this. ST-19 is near the centre of the body, which should have been a safe couple of inches from the gall bladder's usual position. However, the enlargement of the man's organs had shifted his gall bladder, placing the fundus immediately under this acupoint.

The gall bladder's structure is under pressure from the liquid it contains, so that when the organ is punctured it automatically squirts bile into the peritoneal cavity. Bile consists of bile salts, electrolytes, pigments such as bilirubin, cholesterol and other fats. It is also responsible for the elimination of certain waste products from the body. The salts draw fluids from the inner layer of the peritoneum, causing profound irritation that can quickly result in shock and toxic septicaemia.

This condition must be quickly diagnosed and appropriately treated. Mild cases show symptoms within 10 minutes to 6 hours after treatment. Patients feel right upper abdominal pain, which radiates to the right shoulder and scapular region, and nausea, which may cause vomiting. Some cases of peritonitis have developed 1 to 2 days following a treatment; though the perforation itself was tiny, it leaked bile when the patient was digesting a meal. If the gall bladder was already inflamed, a perforation would be much more serious. The patient would experience severe abdominal pain, contraction of abdominal muscles, tachycardia, fast shallow breathing and fever from infection.

What to do in case of gall bladder injury

When you suspect the gall bladder has been injured, even mildly, advise the patient to refrain from eating for several hours. Consuming food will cause the gall bladder to contract, which would push bile into the digestive system and increase the danger of leakage. The patient should be asked to rest. There are some specific herbal medicines that are effective in this case. If the abdominal discomfort does not resolve itself or worsens after several hours of fasting and rest, the patient should be advised to seek medical attention.

Serious cases require hospital care, antibiotics and perhaps surgery to extract bile from the abdominal cavity.

Prevention of gall bladder injury

Prevent gall bladder injury by asking patients their history of abdominal and digestive disorders. If someone reports abdominal pain after eating such fat-laden foods as fried eggs, this is a hint that the gall bladder is inflamed. Further evidence comes from a gentle palpation of the gall bladder's surface projection. This may cause the patient discomfort, so proceed carefully.

When needling points over the surface projection of the gall bladder, we normally perform a shallow insertion in an oblique direction toward the outside of the body. If you think a patient could have an enlarged gall bladder, control the depth of the needle. The maximum safe depth in such a case is dependent on the individual patient's physiology; if unsure, check your reference books for acceptable guidelines. For all patients, stimulation of the needles in these points should be very gentle. In the case of those with enlarged gall bladders, stimulation should be even more restricted, and the needles in this area should be retained for only a short time – no more than 15–20 minutes.

Also, if you suspect enlargement of the organ, it may be advisable to choose points on the patient's left side instead of the right, and select distal rather than local points. During all treatments, observe patients closely and ask them not to change position without your assistance. After the needles have been removed, and the patient is preparing to leave, continue to observe the patient, and ask how he or she is feeling. If you are at all concerned about the possibility of an injury, ask the patient to sit and wait for a few minutes to see whether any symptoms develop.

STOMACH INJURY

The stomach's tough covering makes it the least likely of all the organs to be injured. But because it moves around in the abdominal cavity, and its position is shallow relative to the body's surface, punctures are still possible. Twenty-one cases of acupuncture-related stomach injuries have been reported in the past two decades.

Case study 2.9

A 20-year-old male who felt stomach discomfort after he had been drinking alcohol and eating heavily went for acupuncture. Ten minutes after Ren-12 was needled, the patient felt a severe pain involving the entire abdomen. Ten hours after acupuncture, the young man was admitted to hospital. Doctors found his abdominal muscles rigid with rebound tenderness, and painful to the touch. The white blood cell count was elevated. An X-ray showed a pocket of air under the man's diaphragm. Diagnosis was stomach perforation and peritonitis. An exploratory laparotomy was performed, during which the surgeon found 100 ml of pus in the cavity, as well as a 4×4 cm^2 haematoma on the lesser curvature of the stomach and inflammation of the omenta. A perforation was found near the haematoma, covered by the great omentum. The perforation was repaired, pus and fluids were suctioned out, and drainage tubes inserted. The patient recovered (Xiao 1985).

Related acupoints

See Table 2.1.
When the stomach is full, or in the case of gastroptosis, these points may also be involved: Ren-9, ST-24, ST-25.

Table 2.1

Midline	Ren-13	Ren-12	Ren-11	Ren-10
0.5 cun lateral	KI-20	KI-19	KI-18	KI-17
2 cun lateral	ST-20	ST-21	ST-22	ST-23
4 cun lateral			SP-16	

Discussion of stomach injury

The stomach sits in the upper left quadrant of the peritoneal cavity, immediately behind the front wall of the abdomen and just below the diaphragm, which it touches along part of its length. It is a J-shaped pouch, with its large end directed upward, connected to the oesophagus, and its small end bent to the right, where it terminates at the beginning of the small intestine.

Similar to the gall bladder, the stomach is not a fixed organ but changes size and location according to the person's position and its state of fullness or emptiness. At midfullness, most of the stomach is located in the left hypochondrium with a small portion under the xiphoid process. If the stomach is overextended, it may reach the navel. Its position also varies with the person's age and body type.

The stomach wall itself undergoes peristalsis, contracting as it mixes and digests food. The stomach can move away from a gently probing needle, and even if a tiny perforation is made the stomach is able to contract and close off the wound. This is because the stomach wall consists of three layers of smooth muscle that run in different directions. When irritated, these muscle layers contract according to their direction, so a small hole will be covered over by this defensive mechanism. It is only when a large perforation or tear is made that there is an injury serious enough to cause a haemorrhage and leaking of stomach contents into the cavity, especially after the person has eaten a large meal. The case above is an example of the possible consequences of needling certain points on a patient with an extremely full stomach. The greater curvature of the stomach is normally on the same level as the 10th costal cartilage, and the third lumbar vertebra, but can move 5 cm up or down as it digests food. When the stomach is full, it can be distended downwards so that the greater curvature reaches as far as the umbilicus. This, of course, exposes more points of the Stomach and Ren meridians to potential injury.

Practitioners also need to be aware of the presence of pathological conditions such as gastritis, gastric ulcer, gastroptosis or gastric dilatation. These conditions will change the texture of the stomach wall itself, making it thinner, decreasing its elasticity and weakening its ability to contract. Ulcers or scar tissue also affect the texture and elasticity of the stomach wall, so that it cannot move easily away from a needle or contract to close off a wound.

Because the stomach seems to be well protected by fat and muscle layers, practitioners may be careless about the angle and depth of needle insertion, and too vigorous in stimulation of the needles. You will choose a perpendicular or oblique angle depending on the patient's body type, but you must ensure the needle does not go beyond the stomach muscle and into the cavity. One author reports a single case in which four perforations occurred because the angle, depth and stimulation of a needle were excessive. Each time this incompetent practitioner lifted and thrust the needle he was stimulating, the patient's stomach moved and another wound was inflicted.

What to do in case of stomach injury

If you suspect you have caused an injury, but the patient is not exhibiting any symptoms, ask the person to rest and consume a liquid diet for half a day. Minor discomfort should resolve itself after a couple of days of rest; this could still be related to the patient's original complaint. However, watch for any symptoms of stomach pain, fever or chills, which could be signs of infection. If these occur or worsen, the patient should be sent for medical treatment.

In the case of a serious puncture, within 10 to 20 minutes after treatment the patient will develop extreme pain and vomiting (food sometimes mixed with blood); the abdominal muscles will tighten and guard the area. X-rays will show air below the diaphragm; an operation will be necessary.

Prevention of stomach injury

Before treating stomach points, ask whether the patient has a stomach ulcer, stomach cancer, chronic gastritis, or has eaten a large meal within the past couple of hours. Ulcers are very common. If the answer to any of these questions is yes, be careful in treating local points.

In order to ascertain the correct depth of insertion, and whether to place the needles at a perpendicular or oblique angle, have the patient lie down comfortably face upwards. With your fingers, take a pinch test of the patient's belly fat. If the patient has more muscle than fat on the abdomen, oblique needle placement is best. If there is more fat than muscle, perpendicular needling is fine.

Use the amount of fat in the pinch test as a guide to depth as well. If, for example, the roll of fat is an inch thick between my fingers, I will insert the needle no more than 1.25 cm (half an inch) deep if I'm placing it on the perpendicular angle, and no more than 1.7 cm (two-thirds of an inch) deep if insertion is oblique.

Practitioners want to be sure that the needle stays in the abdominal wall, which includes the layers of skin, fat, muscle and peritoneum. As the fat layer is generally the thickest of these, the pinch test is a good guide to safe insertion depth. This technique is also a useful guide to determining safe depth over any of the major organs – especially liver and intestine – that are accessible through the abdominal wall.

Prevent stomach injury by retaining needles within the abdominal wall, stopping insertion before you feel the empty space that is the peritoneal cavity. If you sense this empty space, withdraw the needle.

INTESTINAL INJURY

Reports of intestinal injury from acupuncture are rare. Two authors who collected statistics on this found 17 and 19 cases respectively (some of which overlapped). In all reported cases, severe complications, including secondary peritonitis, resulted from intestinal content flowing into the peritoneal cavity. Two of these were fatal. One was a case of ileum perforation followed by toxaemia. In the second, the ileum and transverse colon were punctured leading to toxic shock and multiorgan failure.

Case study 2.10

A 38-year-old female had acupuncture to relieve abdominal pain in the umbilical area. After treatment, the pain became worse and the patient began vomiting. She went to hospital about 12 hours after the treatment. The examining physician found signs of peritoneal irritation: guarding and rebound tenderness of the abdomen, and gurgling sounds. An X-ray indicated free air under the diaphragm, and multiple levels of fluid in the intestine.

Diagnosis was an intestinal obstruction and gastroduodenal perforation, with general peritonitis. Surgery was performed, during which a 180° clockwise twist was found at the end of the ileum. The torsion – the cause of the woman's original abdominal pain – had caused a ballooning of a section of the intestine, which was dark red in colour.

The surgeon removed the kink in the ileum and returned it to its proper position. He also found 12 acupuncture marks in the jejunum and ileum, five of which were perforations sufficiently deep to allow intestinal contents to bubble from them. Each of these holes was surgically repaired, and the patient subsequently recovered (Zhao 1978).

Related acupoints

All Stomach, Spleen, Kidney, Gall Bladder, Ren and Extra points located on the anterior of the body below the diaphragm and above the pelvis.

We should be especially careful when needling the following points, because of their location and because they are so frequently used:

ST-21, ST-25, ST-30
Ren-4
SP-13, SP-15.

Discussion of intestinal injury

The small intestine, consisting of the duodenum, jejunum and ileum, is the site where digestion is completed and nutrients are absorbed. It is the portion of the gastrointestinal tract between the pylori sphincter of the stomach and the ileocaecal valve opening into the large intestine. The whole small intestine is positioned in the central and lower portions of the abdominal cavity (Fig. 2.8).

Generally, the jejunum lies more to the left of the navel, and the ileum under the umbilicus and into the right lower abdomen. The diameter of the jejunum is larger and thicker than that of the ileum. The small intestine, except for the duodenum, is supported by mesentery, an apron of connective tissue.

It is important for acupuncturists to understand this portion of the anatomy. Although the attachment of the fan-shaped mesentery to the intestine generally prevents the intestine from becoming twisted or kinked, it also can prevent the intestine from moving away from a probing needle. However, if the intestines are diseased already, there is a twisting or obstruction, or if needle insertion is aggressive, injury is possible.

The small intestine is approximately 2.5 cm wide and 3 m. long in a living person. (It is interesting to note that it is twice as long in a cadaver, when all its muscles are fully relaxed; this is an indication of the strength of muscle activity in the digestive system.) As acupuncturists we must keep in mind that its designation as 'small' is relative only to the large intestine; in reality it takes up a significant amount of space and can therefore be punctured if we are careless in our needle insertion.

The large intestine connects to the bottom end of the ileum, in the lower right section of the abdominal cavity. It consists of the caecum, colon, rectum and anal canal. The colon itself is subdivided into ascending, transverse, descending and sigmoid portions. The large intestine is about 6.5 cm in diameter and 1.5 m long, and a part of the mesentery called the mesocolon supports it along the rear abdominal wall. While the large intestine has little part

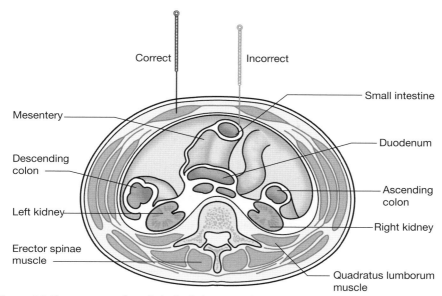

Figure 2.8 Transverse section of the body between the levels of L-3 and L-4. The correct depth of needle placement is in the muscle and fat layers of the abdominal wall. Excessive depth will pierce the intestine.

in digestion, it secretes mucus and absorbs water and electrolytes from the materials that pass into it from the small intestine. It also forms, stores and expels waste from the body – and therefore houses many bacteria.

Similar to the stomach, in a healthy intestine, when a gently probing needle touches the surface, there is enough room for the intestine to move out of the way. But if the intestine is diseased or inflamed by food poisoning, bacterial infection, or a twist or obstruction, its mobility is compromised, leaving it more open to puncture. Also, when there is pathology in the intestine, bacterial action will aerate its contents creating inner pressure and enlarging the intestine. This also inhibits the organ's ability to contract if a needle touches it. In the case of a puncture, the bacteria-laden contents of the intestine will leak out into the abdominal cavity.

Most cases of intestinal injury from acupuncture are caused by one or both of these two factors: the organ is enlarged, or the practitioner has placed a needle too deeply or stimulated it too roughly.

When the ileum of the small intestine is perforated, patients at first seem all right, but quickly develop chemical peritonitis from digestive fluids that have escaped into the abdominal cavity. When the large intestine is perforated, patients rapidly develop bacterial peritonitis, which is life threatening because the large intestine's contents contain toxic bacteria.

What to do in case of intestinal injury

In a mild case, where the surface of the intestine (especially the small intestine) has just been touched by a needle, the symptoms are often vague. There may be some abdominal discomfort, localised under the acupuncture site. The pain will not appear immediately, but develops gradually 4–6 hours after treatment as the leaking intestinal fluids begin to irritate the abdominal cavity and bacteria start to grow. Sometimes it takes as much as 24 hours before the patient experiences abdominal pain, so it can be difficult to make the link between the symptoms and the treatment.

If your patient reports these symptoms to you, and you know you have used acupoints in the intestinal area, suggest that the patient see a physician and let the doctor know that acupuncture may be a factor. Otherwise the patient may have to undergo a huge battery of unnecessary tests.

If you suspect you have accidentally punctured the intestine, instruct the patient to remain in a semireclined position supported by pillows. This will reduce the leakage of waste matter into the cavity. The patient may consume a small amount of liquid, but no solid food. Transport the patient to a hospital, where blood tests and an X-ray will be performed and antibiotics prescribed. In a mild case, the patient should recover without surgery.

With a more serious wound, there will be pain spreading over the entire abdomen, nausea and vomiting, high fever, abdominal guarding and tightness, and air in the abdominal cavity (shown by X-ray). This requires immediate hospitalisation, antibiotics and surgery.

Prevention of intestinal injury

Prevent intestinal injury by obtaining thorough medical histories from your patients. If someone comes for treatment of a stomach ache that has recently arisen and is not chronic, and you suspect the presence of some intestinal pathology, it may be advisable to suggest the patient be checked by a physician first. In the case history above we can see the danger of treating abdominal pain without having a clear idea whether pre-existing disease contraindicates acupuncture. Practitioners should make sure that the patient does not have an acute abdomen – in other words a condition that requires surgery – such as appendicitis or a twisted bowel.

Timing is the key factor in judging whether to treat patients or send them for medical assessment. If abdominal discomfort is acute and has come on suddenly or during a short time, it is best for the patient to seek a medical diagnosis before treating with acupuncture.

If, after having considered these factors, you feel acupuncture would still be helpful, avoid needling abdominal areas around the intestine, and treat points on legs and arms instead. If you see that the patient has scar tissue on the stomach, be alert to the possibility that previous surgery has left adhesions that have glued the intestine to the abdominal wall. This means the intestine will be unable to move away from a needle. Avoid needling on, or even near, scar tissue.

As always when working around vulnerable areas, use gentle technique and be sure the patient doesn't make large or abrupt movements during treatment. In such a sensitive area, leave the needle in for no more than 15 minutes to avoid causing discomfort to the patient. Observe to be sure the patient's movements have not changed the angle or even the depth of the needle. Bending the knees, for instance, can drive an abdominal needle right through the muscle and into an organ.

Use the 'pinch test' to appraise the thickness of the abdominal fat and muscle layers before treating (Fig. 2.9). Place the needle at a depth that is no more than half the distance between your two fingers, and tune in to the sensation to make sure you are not entering 'empty space', in other words into the abdominal cavity. When needling abdominal points, always bear in mind the presence of vital organs and the risk of injury. Awareness prevents accidents.

It is generally best when treating abdominal points to have the patient lie face up rather than on one side, so the intestines don't slosh over to the lower side and move into a risky position. If you must use back points during the same treatment, I recommend dealing with the abdominal points first, then removing these needles and having the patient turn on one side for treatment of the back points.

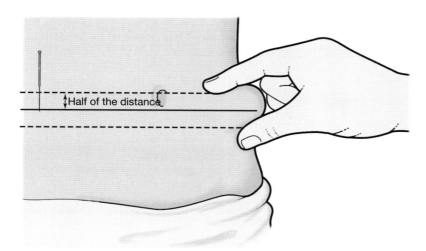

Half of the distance

Figure 2.9 Ascertaining the thickness of abdominal fat and muscle for safe needle placement.

SPLEEN INJURY

The spleen is a very spongy, soft and vulnerable organ in the abdominal cavity. Its pulp contains a great deal of blood for such a small structure, and many vessels run through it. A ruptured or punctured spleen generally results in haemorrhagic shock, followed by secondary peritonitis from the irritation to surrounding tissues from seeping blood.

Case study 2.11

A 35-year-old male had been experiencing vague pain in the left upper abdominal region for 6 months. Over 3 days, the pain worsened, and was accompanied by nausea and vomiting. The patient sought acupuncture treatment. The acupuncturist chose the points SP-16, ST-21 and ST-22, and left the needles in place for 10 minutes. After the needles had been removed, the patient complained the pain in the left upper stomach was worse, and had spread to the entire abdomen. He had also developed severe bloating of the abdomen, thirst, nervousness and shortness of breath. The patient had a history of malaria in childhood.

After the acupuncture treatment, the man was admitted to hospital. An examination found the abdominal muscles to be tender, rigid and distended, and percussion of the area indicated fluid in the abdomen. The patient was rushed into surgery, where an inch-long (2.5 cm) laceration was discovered on his spleen. Nine hundred millilitres of blood were suctioned from the abdominal cavity, and a splenectomy was performed.

Analysis of this case suggests three major factors contributed to this accident. First, the man's bout of malaria had left his spleen enlarged to a point far below the ribcage, so that its surface was directly beneath ST-21. Secondly, the needle was placed too deeply. Then, when the patient took a breath, the needle scratched the spleen causing severe blood loss (Wang et al 1996).

Related acupoints

Left side: ST-21, SP-16, LIV-13, GB-25.

If the spleen is enlarged, the following points can also be involved:

Left side: ST-19, ST-20, SP-15.

Discussion of spleen injury

The spleen is a gland that assists other organs in producing lymphocytes, filtering the blood and destroying old red blood cells. Normally an adult's spleen is the same size as the palm of the hand. It is located posterior and lateral to the stomach, below the diaphragm in the left hypochondrium, covered by the ninth, 10th and 11th ribs (see Fig. 2.7 for surface projection of spleen).

Because it is so well protected, the spleen should be difficult to puncture unless it is enlarged. However, it moves up and down in a range of 2–3 cm with the diaphragm's motion during respiration, and as the stomach expands and contracts with the volume of stomach contents.

There are no acupuncture points on the surface projection of the spleen, but left-side GB-25 and LIV-13 are close to its lower border, so if the needle is inserted incorrectly at an upward angle there is a risk of puncture.

Splenomegaly presents the greatest risk of injury from acupuncture. Many diseases can cause the spleen to enlarge; these include infections such as hepatitis, syphilis, typhoid fever and tuberculosis, various anaemias, blood cancers such as leukaemia, inflammatory diseases, liver ailments such as cirrhosis, cysts and some parasites.

When splenomegaly occurs, the spleen becomes brittle and huge, and its borders may push up the diaphragm, move the stomach outward and even reach the ileum. This makes the spleen accessible through acupuncture points that are normally a safe distance away. In all reported spleen injuries, the organ has been enlarged by 1.5 to 2 times its normal size.

One kind of injury is a tension haematoma, in which the slow bleeding is contained underneath the spleen's capsule. Initially, the patient may not show any sign of injury other than mild distension or discomfort. Two days to 1 week later, the haematoma ruptures, resulting in intraperitoneal haemorrhage.

Symptoms are severe pain, abdominal distension, nausea and vomiting, abdominal guarding and tightness, pallor, thirst, weak pulse, a falling blood pressure and shock. This is a life-threatening medical emergency that calls for immediate blood transfusion and surgery.

What to do in case of spleen injury

If you think your needle has touched the patient's spleen, stop the treatment and remove all the needles. Check pulse and blood pressure several times. If any of the symptoms listed above are present, have the patient transported immediately to a hospital emergency ward. Even if symptoms are mild or vague, or you think the needle just touched the organ briefly before it was withdrawn, you may suggest the patient be examined just to be sure.

Even when the patient has not developed enough symptoms to result in admission to hospital, we still need to bear in mind the possibility of a slow-leaking tension haematoma. At that point, the patient will be monitored by a medical doctor, but the acupuncturist also has a responsibility to ascertain whether any further symptoms have developed and if so, advise the patient to seek medical treatment.

In the case of a rupture, a splenectomy and prophylactic antibiotics are indicated. The spleen is not considered a vital organ in adults. In an infant, it is crucial for the production of red blood cells.

Prevention of spleen injury

Prevent an injury to the spleen by knowing what can cause splenomegaly and asking patients about their history.

Because the enlarged spleen lies next to the stomach and may press against it, the patient may complain of acid reflux, or feel full after eating a small amount or even without having eaten. There may be abdominal pain in the area of the spleen.

Palpate the area to check whether the spleen is enlarged. Keep needles within the abdominal wall. If you sense an empty sensation or elastic resistance below, back off. Needles should also be backed off or even removed if the patient develops a sudden spasmodic cough. This applies to treatment points anywhere on the torso, not just over the spleen.

Watch for three signs of medical emergency: pallor, thirst and pain.

KIDNEY INJURY

Kidney injuries from acupuncture are very uncommon, though not unheard of. Points on the lower back are used daily in a huge variety of treatment situations, but because the muscles in that area tend to be thick it takes a fair degree of incompetence on the part of the practitioner to penetrate right through to the kidney. An author in China has collected only five cases of acupuncture-related kidney injury, and no fatalities have been reported in the literature so far as I have been able to determine. However, if an injury does occur, the consequences are always serious and will require surgery to repair the puncture and stop bleeding, or in severe cases may result in a nephrectomy.

Discussion of kidney injury

In regard to surface projections, the left kidney is 3.5 to 10 cm to the left of the midline of the back, from the lower border of T11 vertebra down to the lower border of L2 vertebra (Fig. 2.10). (The left 12th rib obliquely crosses the

Case study 2.12

A male, 37 years old, sought acupuncture for stomach ache. During the first treatment, the practitioner employed points on the arms and the chest only. For the second and third treatments, points on the kidney region of lower back were added – two needles on the left side and two on the right. Three days after the third treatment, a swelling came up under the muscle in the right kidney region. The patient went to hospital, where he was diagnosed with perinephritis – an inflammation of the tissue surrounding the kidney. A course of antibiotics successfully reduced the inflammation.

However, 10 days later, the patient developed a fever, low back pain and frequent urination, and was admitted to hospital. Antibiotics were continued, and an extraction of 200 ml of blood from the kidney was performed, followed by exploratory surgery. The surgeon found 100 ml of old blood in the renal subcapsular area. A golf-ball-sized lump inside the kidney itself also contained some blood. The bleeding had originated from a fissure in the kidney that was 6–8 cm long, 0.5–1 cm deep. The bleeding had stopped before the surgery, but adhesions had already formed, so the surgeon had to remove the patient's right kidney. The patient recovered (Liu 1957).

Related acupoints

BL-20 – 24, BL-48 – 52
GB-25
Ex. Yao Yan

centre of the left kidney; this is a useful starting point for palpation.) The right kidney is usually half a vertebra lower than the left kidney (1 to 2 cm lower) and situated 3.5 to 10 cm to the right of the midline of the back. In most cases the kidney moves, although only by a distance of one vertebra, according to respiration and body position.

The kidneys are called retroperitoneal organs because they lie outside the abdominal cavity, behind the peritoneum. The kidneys lie closest to the back; very seldom is a kidney injured from the front of the body because the stomach, intestines and liver are in the way. The only real likelihood of kidney injury is through the back in areas where the organ projects closer to the surface.

The points that are the most vulnerable to injury, and which therefore we need to be most cautious about, are: BL-49, BL-50, BL-51 and BL-52. Another group somewhat less risky is: BL-20–24, GB-25 and Ex. Yao Yan. In all cases, excessive depth of needling is the major risk factor.

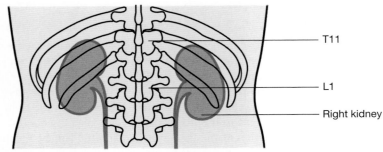

Figure 2.10 Posterior surface projection of the kidneys.

Acupuncturists have to pay attention to the thickness of the fatty and muscular tissue over the kidneys when plotting treatment points. The safe depth of needling in the lower back has, in fact, been suggested by a group of Chinese doctors who performed CT scans on more than 100 patients. Their report says that, regardless of whether the person was overweight or underweight, 'the three acupoints with the least thick fatty tissue in the lower back were: BL-48, BL-49 and BL-50. The tissues averaged a mean depth of 1.01, 1.00 and 1.02 cm respectively. Additionally, the three acupoints with the least thick muscle tissue were BL-48, BL-49 and BL-51, with tissues averaging a mean depth of 3.18, 3.18 and 3.10 cm respectively. The variation in thickness of muscle tissue was much greater than that of fatty tissue' (Lin et al 1998).

We can see that the two groups of points, in fatty and muscle tissue, overlap in BL-48 and BL-49. This warns us that in dealing with these two points we consistently have less room for error before reaching the kidney. BL-50 and BL-51 are slightly different: BL-50 tends to have less fatty tissue around it and BL-51 on average has less muscle tissue. Over all, however, these four points in the kidney region present a risk of injury from mistakes in depth or direction of needle insertion.

Detailed knowledge of anatomy guides practice in choosing the appropriate needle size. Taken together, the fatty tissue and muscle tissue add up to a maximum of 4.02 cm or 40.2 mm. in thickness in most people. Therefore it is important to keep in mind the length of the needles used. Two cun needles are 50 mm long; 3 cun needles measure 75 mm. Normally, for points in the lower back, we use a 2–3 cun needle, depending on the patient's individual body type. So if a 2 cun needle has been inserted to its maximum length, perpendicular to the body, it is likely to have gone through the fat and muscle and possibly have punctured or lacerated the kidney.

What to do in case of kidney injury

If the needles touch only the superficial capsule of the kidney or the shallow part of the renal parenchyma layer surrounding the organ, only small vessels will be ruptured, without a more serious injury to the renal calices or renal pelvis. A puncture to the small vessels would result in loss of only a microscopically detectable quantity of blood cells. Several days' rest should ensure the patient's full recovery. If the deeper, functional structures of the kidney, such as the calices or pelvis, are punctured, blood in the urine will be obvious to the naked eye.

A serious wound would cause leakage of urine into the layer between the kidney and the renal capsule, or even into the surrounding tissues. There may be bruising or swelling on the organ, and subsequent infection. The patient will have a high fever and exhibit symptoms of shock. This may be life threatening and requires immediate treatment.

Injuries may not be noticeable right away. In the case cited above, the blood-filled bruise did not appear until 3 days after the third treatment. If, several days to a week after acupuncture treatment, there is a swelling or pain in the needled area, be alert to the possibility of a kidney injury.

Symptoms of a minor injury are slight backache, muscle rigidity, fatigue and microscopic haematuria. Recovery takes an average of 2 weeks, and may also call for a course of herbs with haemostatic properties, as well as antibiotics.

Severe injuries puncture the renal parenchyma causing haematoma underneath the capsule. Patients feel severe distending pain radiating to the shoulder above, tight lumbar muscles and pain upon touch. A palpable mass at the back may also be evident at the front, and there will be visible haematuria. Send the patient immediately to a physician or the emergency department. If treatment is begun without delay, it may be possible to avoid the need for surgical repair. As long as blood in the urine and the patient's temperature are improving over the course of a few days, surgery may not be necessary. However, leakage of urine or the development of an infection may make an operation inevitable.

Prevention of kidney injury

For the points on the first line of the bladder meridian (BL-20–BL-24) the direction of needle insertion should be oblique and toward the spine, and depth should not be excessive (Fig. 2.11). The spine in this area is well protected by muscle. For the points on the second line of the bladder meridian (BL-48–BL-52) we point the needles in the opposite direction, toward the outside edge of the body, also at an oblique angle and not too deeply.

The average safe depth, depending on the patient's body type, would be 1–1.5 cm at an oblique angle. There may be exceptions when a patient is very heavy or very thin.

Pay attention to the needle sensation (heavy and firm in muscle, then empty, then the elastic resistance of a kidney) and be prepared to back off the needle's depth if you sense empty space – a good principle in general.

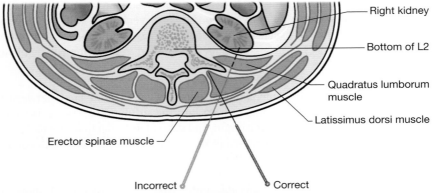

Figure 2.11 Correct and incorrect needling direction for points on the first line of the Bladder meridian. This diagram shows the transverse section of the body between the levels of L2 and L3. To avoid puncturing a kidney, the needle should be angled in the direction of the spine.

Be aware of abnormal kidney locations, as in a 'floating kidney'. Also called a 'moveable kidney', or in medical language ectopia, this is a birth defect in the formation or position of the kidney. The organ could be punctured accidentally when the acupuncturist is not aware that it is situated in a place where it is not normally found. A clue to this possibility would be that such a patient would probably have chronic back pain and chronic urinary system infections. The only way of finding out for sure that a patient has a floating kidney is with an X-ray or ultrasound; therefore this situation must be dealt with by a physician.

BLADDER INJURY

There are very few reports of injuries to the urinary bladder from acupuncture. But because the lower abdomen has many acupoints that are used on a daily basis in treating a wide variety of conditions, there are some factors that deserve attention.

Case study 2.13

An adult male was admitted to hospital for chronic glomerular nephritis. After a week of Western medicine treatment, the patient began to suffer from intermittent gastrointestinal pain. Acupuncture treatment was performed on Ren-4 and Ren-6, followed by moxa treatment.

The gastrointestinal discomfort responded well to this treatment. However, later that night, the patient began to feel nausea and a continuous pain that was localised in centre of the lower abdomen. Physicians examined him and,

continued overpage

knowing that he had had acupuncture earlier in the day, decided to perform a laparotomy. This procedure revealed a perforation at the base of the bladder, coinciding with the level of the acupoint Ren-4. The surgeon also observed a slow, drop-by-drop leakage of urine into the peritoneal cavity. The puncture was surgically repaired and the patient went on to a full recovery (Wang et al 1996).

Related acupoints

Ren-2, Ren-3, Ren-4
KI-11, KI-12, KI-13
ST-28, ST-29, ST-30

Discussion of bladder injury

The urinary bladder is located just behind the pubic symphysis, and in front of the rectum. When empty, it sits in front of the parietal peritoneum, and has the shape of an inverted pyramid. As the bladder fills with urine, its superior surface enlarges and bulges upward into the peritoneal cavity, and the organ becomes more ovoid in shape.

The peritoneum is like a sheath covering the apex of the bladder. Along the midline, these structures are essentially 'glued' together by connective tissue. On the lateral parts of the bladder, the peritoneum is more like a loose covering over the organ. Therefore, when we are needling points on the Ren meridian along the body's centre line, the needle will encounter more resistance in the connection between the peritoneum and the bladder, even though this tissue is thin. In pushing the needle, there is danger of puncturing the bladder. In the lateral areas, on points on the kidney and stomach meridians, the tissue is looser and therefore easier to get through. The bladder can be punctured without our being aware of it.

Another factor of which acupuncturists must be aware is whether the patient's bladder is full or empty. As previously mentioned, a full bladder will be rounded and its apex distended upward into the abdominal cavity, sometimes almost to the level of the umbilicus. When the top of the bladder extends higher than the pubic bone, it becomes vulnerable to injury.

Additional caution is indicated when treating children. The apex of a child's bladder is normally higher than the pubic bone, whether empty or full. Also, children's bladders are always close to the abdominal wall, and there is little or no fat or muscle tissue to protect it. Parents often bring children to an acupuncture clinic for treatment of enuresis. Our primary treatment points for this condition are Ren-2–Ren-4, KI-11–KI-13, as well as SP-6. We must pay particular heed to needle depth and direction when treating children.

What to do in case of bladder injury

During treatment, if a patient is feeling a heavy, distending pain in the lower abdomen, you should suspect that a needle has touched the bladder. Remove the needle immediately. It may be that only the muscle and membrane have been injured and the bladder wall itself has not been perforated. Normally, a minor injury will resolve itself after a few days of rest.

A puncture of the bladder itself will cause bleeding, and leakage of urine into the peritoneal cavity. The toxic wastes contained in urine are irritating to the interior of the peritoneal cavity.

If urine leaks outside the peritoneum, into the surrounding perivesical space, pericystitis will develop. The patient will experience strong pain in the lower abdomen and a distending pain of the rectum and perineum.

Whether the perforation results in urinary seepage inside or outside the peritoneum, antibiotics will be necessary, and possibly surgery as well. Therefore the patient should be sent to a physician or hospital emergency ward as soon as possible. Signs of a perforated bladder are not immediately evident; it may take half an hour to several hours after treatment for symptoms to arise, depending on the rate of urinary diffusion.

Prevention of bladder injury

If you will be treating points in the lower abdomen, it is advisable to ask patients whether they have emptied their bladder recently, and, if they have not, to do so before treatment (Figs 2.12, 2.13). When needling this area, we must be especially careful to insert the needle in a controlled manner. Stimulation of the needle to reach de qi must also be more gentle than usual. The needle should be twirled within a small range of motion, and should not be lifted and thrust as we might do when treating other points. If care is taken

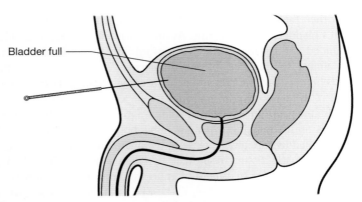

Bladder full

Figure 2.12 Position of needle when bladder is full.

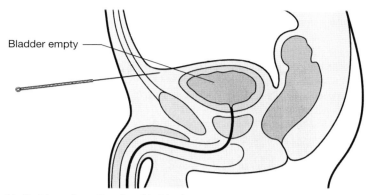

Bladder empty

Figure 2.13 Position of needle when bladder is empty.

in manipulation of the needle, even if injury occurs it will be a small puncture and not a large hole or laceration.

In addition, needles should be retained in these points for only 10 minutes or so, because urine will continue to accumulate in the bladder during treatment. As the patient begins to feel an urgent need to urinate, restlessness and movement increase the possibility of puncture.

In many countries, acupuncture is a common and very effective treatment for patients suffering from retention of urine. This can occur after a stroke, postsurgically, as a result of irritation after a pelvic examination or as a side-effect of some medications. Paradoxically, having a full bladder makes it difficult to treat urinary retention! In addition to the cautions outlined above, it is important in this case to insert needles in these vulnerable points at an angle that is quite shallow relative to the surface of the body – generally no more than 30°.

This also applies when treating children, especially those less than 10 years of age. The angle of needle insertion should be closer to about 15°– so that the needle is almost lying flat. In older or larger children the angle should still be no more than 30°.

References

Brettel HF 1981 Akupunktur als Todesursache. München Medizinische Wochenschrift 123:97-98

Chen Hanwei et al 1963 Discussing acupuncture injuries to organs inside the abdominal cavity. Chinese Medicine Journal 4:26

Feng Lizhong 1965 To avoid injuring organs, careful examination is needed before stomach acupuncture. Medical Journal for Middle Level Practitioners 9:585

Halvorsen TB, Anda SS, Naess AB et al 1995 Fatal cardiac tamponade after acupuncture through congenital sternal foramen. The Lancet 345:1175

Jin Bairen 1987 One case report of pneumothorax by needling SI-13. Shanghai Journal of Acupuncture 3:45

Jaung-Geng Lin, Li Tsai-Chung, Li Hsu-Jan, et al 1998 Determination of safe needling depth via CT-scan studies of tissue thicknesses at acupoint locations of the lower back. American Journal of Acupuncture 26(2/3):121-127

Kataota H 1997 Cardiac tamponade caused by penetration of an acupuncture needle into the right ventricle. Journal of Thoracic and Cardiovascular Surgery 114:674-676

Kirchgatterer A, Schwarz CD, Holler E et al 2000 Cardiac tamponade following acupuncture. Chest 117(5):1510-1511

Liu Shiyi 1957 Injury of the renal region caused by acupuncture. Medical Journal for Middle Level Practitioners 10:637

Liu Xinji 1981 Four cases of acupuncture accident in treatment of patients with schizophrenia. Journal of Neuropsychosis (China) 5:317

McCormick WF 1981 Sternal foramina in man. American Journal of Forensic Medical Pathology 2:249-252

Mazal DA, King T, Harvey J et al 1980 Bilateral pneumothorax after acupuncture. New England Journal of Medicine 302(24):1365-1366, cited in Rosted, P 2004 Adverse reactions after acupuncture: a review no. 2. Online. Available: http://users.med.auth.gr/~karanik/english/articles/adverse1.html

Peuker E, Gronemeyer D 2001 Rare but serious complications of acupuncture: traumatic lesions. Acupuncture in Medicine 19(2):103-108

Rosted P 2004 Adverse reactions after acupuncture: a review no. 2. Online. Available: http://users.med.auth.gr/~karanik/english/articles/adverse1.html

Rotchford JK 2004 Adverse events of acupuncture. Online. Available: www.medicalacupuncture.com/aama_marf/journal/Vol. 11_2/adverse.html

Wang Xiuying Han Youdong, Zhang Xiaolian et al 1996 Acupuncture accidents: their prevention and cure. Shandong Science and Technology Publishing House, Jinan

White A, Ernst E 2001 Adverse events associated with acupuncture reported in 2000. Acupuncture in Medicine 19(2):136-139

Wright RS, Kupperman JL, Liebhaber MI 1991 Bilateral tension pneumothorax after acupuncture. Western Journal of Medicine 154(1):102-103, cited in Rosted P 2004 Adverse reactions after acupuncture: a review no. 2. Online. Available: http://users.med.auth.gr/~karanik/english/articles/adverse1.html

Xiao Xuetang 1985 One case report of stomach perforation by acupuncture. Chinese Rural Medicine Journal 1:9

Zhao Jiuxiang 1978 Acupuncture treatment injury to small intestine; case misdiagnosed as duodenal perforation. Guang Xi Barefoot Doctor Medical Journal 4:34

Zhou Jianwei 1995 Acupuncture injuries and safe needling techniques for dangerous points. Sichuan Science and Technology Publishing House, Chengdu

Infection and disease transmission

3

NEEDLING INFECTION

Postacupuncture infection is easy to avoid; if it does occur it can be minor or quite serious – even fatal. There are two types: a bacterial infection after needling, and the transmission of viruses such as HIV and hepatitis. The latter will be dealt with in a separate section.

Here, we take a brief look at a selection of reported cases that illustrate different aspects of the risk of infection from acupuncture.

Case studies

A 59-year-old man was referred for acupuncture treatment for chronic lower back pain, which had become worse 3 weeks after knee replacement surgery on both legs. A series of three weekly treatments took place, during which disposable sterile needles were placed in points superficial to the muscle fascia around the knees, including KI-10 and BL-40. Three weeks later, the man developed pain in his left knee, and cultures of the fluid subsequently drained from the surgical wound were positive for *Staphylococcus aureus* (Braverman & Prieto 1998).

In another case, a 33-year-old man began to experience hip pain after he played a hockey game. He was diagnosed with a muscle strain and given non-steroidal anti-inflammatory medication. At the time, he was also running a slight fever but this was not treated. When the patient's hip pain did not improve, he

continued overpage

continued

went for acupuncture treatments, involving needles on his hips, legs and feet. He noticed at the time that his skin had not been cleaned by the practitioner before treatment. Despite further treatment by his own physician, the man's pain continued to get worse; he developed fevers, night sweats and vomiting, as well as multiple patches of red, swollen skin on his arm, shoulder and foot. He was admitted to hospital, where blood cultures yielded *S. aureus* (Leavy 2002).

Finally, a 56-year-old diabetic man fell and hurt his right flank, though the skin was not broken. When his discomfort did not resolve, he went for a course of acupuncture treatments over 10 days. After these were completed, the patient developed a painful swelling on his right flank, chills and fever, and an elevated white blood cell count. In hospital, a CT scan revealed a 10 cm abscess on the right-side back muscle and abdominal wall. *Klebsiella pneumoniae* bacteria were found in the blood and pus samples (Cho et al 2003).

In all three cases, the patients recovered fully after appropriate treatment with drainage and antibiotics, though in the case of the man with the knee replacements the affected prosthesis had to be surgically removed and replaced.

Related acupoints

Theoretically, any point.

Discussion of needling infection

It goes without saying that antiseptic practice by acupuncturists is essential. But these three cases illustrate the fact that certain patients are at greater than normal risk for needling infection, and that practitioners must be even more rigorous in ensuring a sterile environment when treating such people. These include those with:

- heart valve surgery or knee or hip replacements
- diabetes
- myocardial damage from previous infection of the heart muscle
- suppressed immune systems from previous infections, or from use of antirejection medications or high doses of steroids
- any open wounds.

As we can see, any situation in which blood circulation is impeded, healing is slow or the immune system is suppressed raises the risk of opportunistic infection. In the cases above, although it is impossible to prove that the needling introduced bacteria into the patients, this could have been a factor, especially where it was known that the practitioner did not first clean the skin.

There is potential for introducing infection at every step of acupuncture. The first is the needle itself. A needle that is reused without proper sterilisation is an obvious source of bacteria. But a clean needle or even an unused disposable needle can be contaminated through improper storage, such as leaving a package open for a few days. These are major sources of acupuncture-related infection. Another risk factor is lack of cleanliness of the practitioner's hands, skin or fingernails. And the patient's own skin, especially around the acupoint, needs to be cleaned in order to avoid infection. Finally, when the needle is withdrawn, until the hole in the skin is fully closed it should not be touched by anything other than a sterile swab. In one reported case, a needling site on a patient's finger was infected when he used his own unclean hand to wipe off a drop of blood. This introduced a bacterium that led to a serious bone infection and a permanent disability in that finger.

We must remember that the skin is one of the body's natural defences; any wound, even a tiny perforation by an acupuncture needle, breaks this defence and can allow contaminants to be introduced into the body. If the patient has a robust immune system, this would probably result, at worst, in a mild, localised infection. But a severe case could set off a systemic infection in the whole body. Infections most commonly associated with acupuncture reported in the literature are: localised abscess, pyoderma, pleuraempyema, peritonitis, epidural abscess, cellulitis (a spreading bacterial infection in the skin), endocarditis, myositis, suppurative arthritis, osteomyelitis and septicaemia. This last, if not caught in time, can affect the heart and brain and rapidly lead to death.

The specific bacteria responsible for these infections include: *Staphylococcus*, *Streptococcus*, *Pneumococcus*, *Pseudomonas* and a large group of organisms that cause such serious conditions as gangrene and tetanus.

What to do in case of needling infection

Signs of infection vary with the type of bacteria involved, but symptoms they have in common are: redness, swelling, pain and tenderness, a sensation of heat and possibly fever. Of course, a patient with a suspected infection should be referred to a physician, or even a hospital emergency department if symptoms are serious. Normally, the doctor will order blood tests, cultures of pus, joint fluid or phlegm, and urine samples to determine what kind of infection is present and which is the most useful antibiotic to prescribe for treatment. If appropriate, the doctor may begin antibiotic therapy even before the lab results are in. When infection has progressed beyond the local stage, antibiotics may be given intravenously.

Chinese medicine has a panoply of herbs that have been shown to be effective in dealing with infection, including: honeysuckle flower (jin yin hu), isatis leaf (da qing ye), isatis root (ban lan gen), dandelion (pu gong ying), wild chrysanthemum flower (ye ju hua), patrinia (bai jiang cao) and Yedo violet (zi hua di ding). A qualified practitioner or herbalist must choose which of these to use in correct proportion with various other herbs in a decoction tailored to the individual patient's specific needs.

Herbs with antibiotic properties may be used in combination with Western antibiotics, or on their own if the infection is not too severe. The decision depends on the patient's condition, the stage of the infection and the practitioner's clinical experience and knowledge.

Prevention of needling infection

A responsible acupuncturist will maintain stringent sterilisation procedures and aseptic techniques. In some jurisdictions there are clear regulations that mandate the use of single-use, disposable needles only. But, in others, practitioners commonly reuse needles either for economic reasons or because they are working in places where there are no regulations governing their practice.

A case in Quebec, Canada, in 2004 exemplifies the importance of sterile needles. Nearly 1200 patients were advised by health authorities to be tested for HIV and hepatitis after it was found that their acupuncturist had been reusing needles and was disinfecting but not sterilising them. Although Quebec is one of the provinces in which acupuncture is regulated, this person had been practising TCM, unlicensed, for 25 years before someone alerted the registrar.

In response to this case, British Columbia's regulatory body, the College of Traditional Chinese Medicine Practitioners and Acupuncturists, immediately adopted a regulation requiring all of its members, including those who had been using autoclaving or other sterilisation practices in the past, to use only disposable needles. Even where regulations are in place, to ensure public safety it is imperative that colleges enforce these rules and that schools of TCM make a point of teaching students aseptic techniques.

Besides the needles, storage jars for cotton balls, tweezers, etc. must be cleaned regularly. Use a squeeze or pump bottle to dispense lubricants, to avoid contamination. Never refill the dispenser without cleaning the bottle first. The container for alcohol should also be cleaned out and its contents replaced regularly; the volatile part of alcohol evaporates leaving only water, which is a breeding ground for bacteria.

Between 2000 and 2002, more than 30 patients of one practitioner came down with confirmed or suspected cases of *Mycobacterium* abscessus, a skin disease characterised by painful, pus-filled bumps that can take months of antibiotic treatment to cure. The practitioner is alleged to have reused disposable needles, and may have stored them in contaminated solutions or used non-sterile solutions to clean patients' skin. *Mycobacterium* abscessus can live and thrive in disinfectants (Gray 2004).

To ensure that sterile conditions are maintained, practitioners must wash their hands with soap and water or a waterless hand rub before treating each patient. The patient's skin around the needling sites must be swabbed with properly stored alcohol, using a sterile cotton ball. After needles are removed, the hole should not be touched by either the practitioner's or the patient's hands for at least a couple of hours, until it is fully closed. The needle site should also be kept dry, so the patient should not shower, bathe or go swimming until the holes have sealed. Although such infections are rare in countries where water supplies are clean, they often occur in regions with more pollution or contaminated water.

Governing bodies such as colleges of TCM and acupuncture are likely to have their own regulations regarding proper aseptic procedures. Those who are practising in unregulated jurisdictions, or who want detailed guidelines, can consult the excellent 'Clean Needle Technique Manual' developed by the National Acupuncture Foundation in the United States in consultation with the Center for Disease Control in Atlanta.[1]

If a patient shows signs of any pre-existing infection, open wound or skin irritation around an acupoint, avoid needling in this area. The treatment can break the skin's line of defence and transmit infection more deeply into the body. Use alternative points.

As mentioned earlier, some people who have heart valve abnormalities, other heart or lung problems or knee or hip replacements are at greater risk for infection. Because the infective consequences are so severe, these patients are often given antibiotics before dental or surgical procedures as a preventive measure. The question arises: is this necessary before acupuncture? In my experience, prophylactic antibiotics are not necessary, but when treating such patients we must be doubly careful to use sterile procedures at each step, from cleaning the skin to treating the holes after needles are withdrawn. Close follow-up is also necessary, so that any signs of infection can be caught early and treated by the patient's physician.

DISEASE TRANSMISSION BY ACUPUNCTURE – A DISCUSSION OF HIV AND HEPATITIS

This issue warrants some extra discussion because of the serious consequences of transmission of diseases such as HIV–AIDS or hepatitis. It is of such public concern that many people avoid acupuncture because they worry about the risk of disease transmission through needles.

This should be of equal concern to acupuncturists. So far, surprisingly, there is only one reported case of acute HIV infection that the literature categorises as 'possibly' linked to acupuncture, because the previously healthy 17-year-old male patient had no history of sexual intercourse, blood transfusion, haemophilia, intravenous drug use or other risk factors, but had been given acupuncture once a week for 6 weeks (Vittecoq et al 1989).

Hepatitis B is more easily transmitted by needle sticks than is HIV, but as a blood-borne virus transmitted in the same way as HIV, it is a good cautionary model that reminds practitioners of the potential danger. Literature reviews describe outbreaks of acupuncture-related hepatitis B in the United States, Israel, the United Kingdom and Europe. None of these cases was linked to disposable needles that had been properly stored and used for that patient only.

In order to provide the necessary reassurance, it is a good idea to explain to all new patients that you are registered and qualified to practise acupuncture, and that you always use one-time-only disposable needles. In addition to using the sterile techniques outlined earlier, practitioners should be sufficiently focused on what they are doing to notice whether a needle has accidentally touched the patient's hair, clothing, pillow or elsewhere on the skin before insertion. If so, the needle should be discarded and a fresh one used.

It is not uncommon for a needle to fall out of a point. Never reinsert the same needle. Replace it with a new one. Attention to such tiny details prevents bigger problems.

SELF-PROTECTION FOR PRACTITIONERS

One of my colleagues has related an incident that shows how easily an acupuncturist can be injured, with potentially serious consequences. She was treating an HIV-positive patient for back pain, needling SI-3. During insertion, the patient's hand jumped, causing the needle to prick the practitioner's finger. The acupuncturist promptly washed and disinfected her hands, removed the rest of the patient's needles and ended the treatment, after which she went immediately to a nearby hospital, which fortunately has a specialty in HIV–AIDS. Because the injury had caused blood to be drawn from the practitioner but not the patient, specialists assessed the case as borderline high risk, and prescribed antiretroviral therapy. These drugs have side-effects such as fatigue and nausea, which were relieved by treatment with Chinese herbs and acupuncture. Eight months after the accident, the HIV tests were negative and the practitioner is still in good health.

There are several reasons such a self-injury can occur; for one, the patient's position on the table has not been properly thought out and the treatment area is not sufficiently exposed. If the practitioner cannot see the skin properly when needles are inserted or withdrawn, a self-inflicted puncture wound can easily occur. This once happened to me when I was trying to avoid disturbing a patient whose lower body was disabled by an accident. In trying to reach the back of the knee, I was attempting to work in a confined space and an awkward angle between the limb and the bed. In retrospect, I should have turned the patient on to one side.

Sometimes a practitioner who is distracted by conversation with the patient, a question from a family member or the ringing telephone will momentarily lose focus while putting in a needle. If a patient unexpectedly moves, for example, while you're doing ear acupuncture, you can drive the needle right through the ear lobe and into your thumb.

When you are running behind schedule and trying to catch up by rushing through needle insertion, an accident is more likely.

If you are treating someone you know is infected with HIV or hepatitis, schedule the treatment so that you have enough time to proceed with extra care and attention to insertion and withdrawal of the needles. Brace your opposite hand on the skin to hold it still and taut while you insert needles, and ask the patient not to move. Take your hands away from the point right away, in case the patient shifts position unexpectedly.

As you are withdrawing needles, transfer them two or three at a time to your sharps container, rather than piling them all into a small dish and transferring them all at once. The more needles are near your hand, the greater the risk of puncture. Also, the sharps container should not be allowed to get more than half full, to avoid having needles pop back up as you are trying to stuff them in.

Ensure that the patient's clothing is pulled back far enough to allow you a clear view of the treatment area without having to get into an awkward posture.

Cotton balls used to wipe points after treatment should be large enough to absorb any blood without allowing it to touch your skin.

If you have a cut on your hand, dress it or wear a surgical glove to protect yourself as well as the patient. If you have any infection on your hand or fingers, it is advisable to cancel appointments and close your clinic for a couple of days to avoid transmitting bacteria or viruses to your patients.

Occasionally, a needle will drop on to the treatment bed linen. Be careful when changing sheets; don't sweep your hands over them, but hold them up by the edges and shake them out so that any lost needles will drop to the floor where they can be swept up.

If you do sustain a puncture wound, use iodine and alcohol to disinfect the wound right away. Report the circumstances of the injury to your own physician or at the emergency ward, where the risk of disease transmission can be assessed.

In the case of hepatitis, prevention is obviously preferable, when possible. Hepatitis A can be transmitted by close physical contact with an infected person; hepatitis B and C viruses are usually spread by blood-to-blood contact, although the risk of acquiring hepatitis C through acupuncture is relatively small. For your protection and that of your patients, consult with your physician or health unit about getting a hepatitis vaccination.

As in most health care professions, acupuncturists are vulnerable to back injuries from moving patients between wheelchairs and treatment tables, for example. There are many written resources you can consult to protect your neck and back.

Protection of the practitioner in terms of social, legal and ethical issues is discussed in Section Two.

Notes

1. Clean needle technique manual, National Acupuncture Foundation, AOM Alliance, 6405 43rd Ave Ct NW, Ste. B, Gig Harbor, WA 98335 USA; phone: 253-851-6896; fax: 253-851-6883; website: www.aomalliance.org.

References

Braverman SE, Prieto RL 1998 Wound infection after total knee arthroplasty and acupuncture: case report and survey of medical acupuncturists. Medical Acupuncture, 13:2, a Journal for Physicians by Physicians accessed on line http://www.medicalacupuncture.com/aama_marf/journal/vol13.2journalindex.html

Cho Yong Pil, Jang HJ, Kim JS et al 2003 Retroperitoneal abscess complicated by acupuncture: case report. Journal of Korean Medical Science 18:756-757

Gray J 2004 Class-action suit to proceed against acupuncturist. The Globe and Mail March 2:A12

Leavy BR 2002 Apparent adverse outcome of acupuncture. Journal of American Board of Family Practice 15(5):246-248

Vittecoq D, Mettetal JF, Rouzioux C et al 1989 Acute HIV infection after acupuncture treatments. New England Journal of Medicine 320(4):250-251

Abnormal reaction to acupuncture

4

NEEDLE FAINTING

Surveys of practitioners in Australia and the United Kingdom list needle fainting as the most common adverse effect associated with acupuncture. It can happen during treatment or even as long as several hours after the needles have been withdrawn. Some patients have been known to faint *before* acupuncture!

Case study 4.1

This case is from my own working notes. I was once invited to speak about traditional Chinese medicine at one of the regular cultural events organised by the Canada–China Friendship Association. The workshop was held in a meeting room of moderate size. After my talk, a woman asked whether I would do a demonstration of acupuncture, showing how the needle goes through the skin, how to stimulate the needle, etc. An older man volunteered to be my 'guinea pig' for the demonstration. I put the needle in, and after a few minutes, during which I did some gentle manipulation, I removed the needle.

At this point, another of the audience members asked what kind of side-effects could be expected from acupuncture. I replied that if acupuncture were performed by a properly trained practitioner there was little or no danger. But occasionally, a patient might pass out. The words were hardly out of my mouth before my volunteer started to look a bit wobbly, pale and sweaty.

In addition to the power of suggestion, several factors combined to make this man feel unwell: the room was small, stuffy and airless, there were at least 40 people crammed into it and the man had never had acupuncture before. I had chosen LI-4 – a point that responds quickly with a strong sensation – in retrospect a misjudgement on my part.

Fortunately I had an intern on hand who quietly revived our volunteer patient by getting him into fresh air, giving him a drink of warm water and performing acupressure while I carried on with the session. The man had fully recovered after a few minutes; I didn't quite dare ask him to describe to the audience his experience of de qi.

Related acupoints

LI-4, LI-10, LI-11, LI-15
ST-9
SI-11, SI-13
TB-3, TB-5
GB-20, GB-21, GB-34

Theoretically, any point can cause needle fainting, but this group collectively has the highest rate of fainting associated with it. The reason is that these points are quick to produce de qi, and the needle sensation is strong.

Discussion of needle fainting

Needle fainting is one of the common vasodepressor syncopes of reflex fainting. The process is that strong acupuncture stimulation combined with nervousness and fear make the blood vessels dilate, via the vagus nerve reflex.

Because the whole body's peripheral vessels dilate, not enough blood can get back to the heart. The resulting reduction in cardiac output causes a temporary drop in blood pressure; this means a reduction of oxygen getting to the brain, and the person faints. Auricular points have a greater chance than body points of causing needle fainting, because a branch of the vagus nerve travels to the ear and therefore the vagus nerve reflex is more likely to be triggered.

Some people casually describe acupuncture fainting as shock, but this is not medically accurate. Shock occurs when major blood loss, inadequate heart function or excessive vasodilation causes severe, prolonged low blood pressure. When the body's cells are deprived of circulation for too long, they are irreversibly damaged; organ failure and death can result.

In shock, the signs of blood pressure drop are clearly evident, severe and long lasting. The major early symptom of needle fainting is lightheadedness, so the most likely possible injury is from a fall.

Needle fainting is most likely to occur in patients who have never had acupuncture before, are fearful of needles, have come for acupuncture on an empty stomach, are dehydrated from perspiring heavily after physical labour, or already have a weak constitution from illness and having spent a lot of time in bed. It can also happen when the practitioner's stimulation techniques of lifting and turning the needles are too aggressive, when electrical stimulation is set too high, or too suddenly, and when the practitioner uses too many needles on a patient who is being treated for the first time.

Patients will usually recover from needle fainting quickly, smoothly and with no lasting effects, but this depends on the patient's constitution and correct management by the practitioner. However, it is easily preventable.

What to do in case of needle fainting

The patient will feel lightheaded or dizzy, and will be pale in the face. There may be nausea, yawning and discomfort in the upper stomach. Some patients will complain of heart palpitations. If the situation deteriorates, the patient may experience blurring of vision, vomiting, sweating and general weakness. Some patients will experience a rapid loss of consciousness; if standing, they will fall. The pulse will be weak and blood pressure can drop. Normally the whole episode from onset to recovery is over in a few minutes, but in rare cases it takes people a couple of hours for symptoms to subside, and the person feels tired and unable to carry on with their regular workload for the rest of the day.

If a patient begins to feel dizzy and lightheaded and starts to yawn, remove all needles right away. Take away the patient's pillows and elevate the legs and feet to speed up recovery by increasing blood flow to the heart and brain. Loosen any tight clothing around the person's neck, and open a window to bring in fresh air. Offer hot water or, even better, warm tea. Check blood pressure. Use your fingernail to apply acupressure to these four points: Du-26,

PC-6, ST-36 and Du-25. With prompt first aid, most people will recover in 3 to 5 minutes. If after 5 minutes the patient's condition deteriorates, especially if there is loss of consciousness, a heart or brain condition may be a factor. It is best not to take chances. Call an ambulance.

Prevention of needle fainting

For patients who are very weak from pre-existing conditions, or who have a serious phobia about needles, you may choose not to do any needling on a first visit. You can employ other therapies such as acupressure or moxibustion. In addition, you can give a reassuring explanation of what to expect in acupuncture, and demonstrate the technique using a very small needle on either yourself or someone who is accompanying the patient.

Normally, when I needle people who are very nervous, I do two things to reduce the discomfort of insertion. One is to use a thumbnail to press firmly on the acupoint, and ask the patient to cough. At that moment, I use my other hand to quickly pop the needle into place. The patient will almost never feel the needle going in, which will help the person relax as the rest of the needles are inserted. Another useful technique is to ask the patient to make an 'O' with each index finger and thumb, and at the count of three to press the nails of the index fingers into the flesh just behind each thumbnail; at that exact moment the needle can be placed. This is not just a technique of distraction; the thumbs are connected to several major meridians, and the resulting energy flow will help the patient to relax. But timing is everything; like an orchestra conductor you have to 'cue' the patient and be ready with your needle.

Obviously, when treating a nervous or weak patient it is wise to use fewer needles, and keep stimulation to a minimum.

A patient who is coming for acupuncture and is sweating from physical exertion should be asked to drink some water and rest for a few minutes before the treatment begins.

During treatment, do not leave the patient unattended. Observe the person closely and ask how he or she is feeling. A person who is not familiar with the normal sensations of acupuncture may not be able to distinguish between sensations of energy flow and the early symptoms of fainting. Close observation will enable you to take prompt action if necessary.

In very rare cases, a patient who has not passed out during the treatment may start to feel lightheaded and ill after all the needles have been removed. When your clinical instincts tell you that a particularly nervous or weak person is at risk of a delayed case of needle fainting, it is a good idea to ask the patient to sit in your waiting room for a few minutes, and perhaps have some warm water, before going home. Then if the patient starts to exhibit fainting symptoms you are still available to assist. Caution is certainly indicated if the patient will be driving home alone.

Over the years I have noticed that more cases of fainting occur in big, hearty-looking males than in small, delicate women! I can only speculate that stronger adrenal response in men makes them more vulnerable to fainting. In any case, it is a good reminder to the practitioner that our judgements of people's health and robustness should be based more on internal factors such as their energy, and not only on their external appearance.

MANIC OUTBURST

Case study 4.2

In one case in China, a patient was treated for a lower back injury with acupuncture on the point Du-26. After the needle had been in for 15 minutes with strong stimulation, the patient began laughing uncontrollably. To control this outburst, the practitioner needled PC-6, LI-4, LIV 3 and the Ex. Shi Xuan on the fingertips. Five minutes later the patient calmed down but felt exhausted (Hao 1986).

Related acupoint

Du-26

Discussion of manic outburst

The cause of this phenomenon is not clearly understood, but a study of the research reveals a couple of possibilities. It has been proven that acupuncture has an effect on brain chemistry. We don't know exactly how this happens, or which specific neurotransmitters may be involved, but it is a reasonable assumption that a change in the level of some chemical in the brain can trigger a manic outburst.

The second possibility is that the insertion of the needle itself can cause enough stimulation or surprise in sensitive individuals to set off a sort of startle reaction or fight-or-flight response. Whichever theory is correct, a manic outburst will occur only in a person who is suggestible, easily overstimulated by environmental factors or psychologically fragile. The person may become hyperactive, or begin laughing hysterically.

From the viewpoint of Chinese medicine, Du-26 is a powerful point. The Du meridian enters the brain, and in the case above the strong stimulation opened the meridian too suddenly, disturbing the patient's emotional balance.

What to do in case of manic outburst

Since Chinese medicine would see manic outburst as related to Liver qi stagnation, we would regulate the qi with acupuncture or moxa, or a herbal patent medicine called 'Xiao Yao San' ('Relieve Liver Qi Stagnation') in a pill or decoction form. Try to calm the patient down with reassuring words and offer a warm drink. If the patient's mania is uncontrollable – an extremely rare manifestation – it is advisable to refer the person to a physician or hospital emergency ward, where a psychiatrist can be consulted.

Prevention of manic outburst

When working on points on the Governing Vessel, which includes many powerful and sensitive points such as Du-20 and Du-26, keep the needle depth shallow, and stimulation very gentle. It is often easy for the practitioner to tell which patients have a tendency to be suggestible, easily overstimulated or anxious, so do gentle treatments on these on all meridians and points.

Du-26 is commonly used to treat acute lower back pain. Increase stimulation gradually at this point, and stop when the patient senses a loosening in the lower back.

INTRACRANIAL HAEMORRHAGE

When we speak of intracranial haemorrhage, this does not mean an injury caused by a needle puncture, as in subarachnoid haemorrhage. It refers to patients with a history of other vascular disease such as high blood pressure or atherosclerosis. In these cases, acupuncture can indirectly induce a brain haemorrhage.

Case study 4.3

This 59-year-old male had a history of chronic hypertension. He had a stroke, and was in hospital for 21 days before his condition was stable enough to go home. A few days later, he began acupuncture treatment for poststroke rehabilitation. The first two treatments left the man feeling well. On the third treatment, Ex. Tai Yang, Du-20 and GB-20 were chosen. During this treatment, the patient complained of a headache and sweating. The practitioner removed all the needles immediately. However, the patient started to vomit. Thirty minutes later he lapsed into a coma, and developed urinary incontinence. After emergency treatment in hospital, the man's left pupil was enlarged. A lumbar puncture revealed a considerable quantity of blood in the cerebrospinal fluid. The diagnosis was intracranial haemorrhage.

In surgery, 35 ml of blood was drained from an intracranial haematoma and a tracheotomy was performed. But the patient died of circulatory and respiratory failure 4 days later.

The author's analysis of this case is that the stimulation of acupuncture induced the man's blood pressure to rise, triggering a rupture of an intracranial blood vessel (Zhou et al 1985).

Related acupoints

GB-4, GB-5, GB-20
Du-20, Du-25, Du-26
Ex. Tai Yang, and all points on the skull
12 Well points (both sides): LU-11, PC-9, HT-9, SP-1, LIV-1, KI-1

Discussion of intracranial haemorrhage

In 70% of the cases of intracranial haemorrhage related to high blood pressure, the bleeding is located in the basal ganglia, which are specialised, paired masses of grey matter deep inside the cerebrum. Within these ganglia, bleeding most commonly occurs in the internal capsule around the lentiform nucleus (capsuloganglionic haemorrhage).

There can also be haemorrhaging from the external capsule and the putamen; this bleeding will compress the internal capsule. The remaining 30% of hypertension-related intracranial haemorrhages occur either under the cerebral cortex, or from vessels in the thalamus, pons, cerebellum or the ventricles. These are all vital parts of the brain, so any damage or bleeding in these areas is life threatening.

The choice of points plays a strong role in indirectly inducing cranial haemorrhage. Some of the points listed above have, in themselves, a tendency to raise blood pressure, and are therefore useful in treating people with shock or hypotension. However, they can be dangerous in someone whose blood pressure is already elevated. A study of 24 cases of low blood pressure, in which Du-25 was used for treatment, resulted in significant improvement in 14 cases and some improvement in 10 (Shi 1987). It is clear that this point has a strong influence on blood pressure.

Du-20 has a similar effect, which has been shown in experiments. This is a situation in which it is imperative to know the patient's history of any high blood pressure or vascular disease.

A second set of points – those located on the head – present a risk because of their proximity to certain small arteries inside the brain. Needling these surface points may cause arterial spasms, possibly resulting in rupture of one of these vessels. If treating a person with a migraine, we must be absolutely certain the headache is not caused by high blood pressure. Among the most commonly used skull points, and therefore the ones related to reported haemorrhages, are GB-4, GB-5 and GB-20, and Ex. Tai Yang.

Points on the tips of the extremities, such as the 12 Well points next to the finger and toenails, are far away from the brain. But they are very sensitive to pain, and the nervousness that some extremely sensitive and reactive people feel when these points are treated may be enough to raise blood pressure. This would be an issue only in a person with pre-existing disease such as atherosclerosis or hypertension.

When some sensitive points such as those listed above are needled, the stimulation sends a bioelectrical pulse into the reticular structure of the brain stem. The brain stem responds with a reflex excitation, especially through the sympathetic nervous system, which causes many peripheral arteries to contract. The increased resistance to blood flow elevates blood pressure.

In a patient with hypertension or atherosclerosis, or both, there will already be deposits of fatty plaque, and damage to the vessel's walls from excessive turbulence of blood flow where the small arteries of the brain branch off at right angles from the larger vessels (Fig. 4.1). These factors create poor circulation through constricted and brittle arteries, and make these spots more susceptible to rupture.

When there is a haemorrhage, there is little room in the skull to allow the tissue to expand, so blood pressure can quickly increase with potentially fatal results. In general, more than half the people who have large haemorrhages die within a few days. People with small haemorrhages, as long as treatment is immediate, usually recover to a remarkable degree.

Ear seeds or auricular acupuncture are not generally the first choice in treating high blood pressure, but acupuncturists have been known to try this. Many of these treatments have been successful, but in some cases blood pressure was actually raised rather than lowered. The cause is unclear. One theory is that the ear branch of the vagus nerve could send an impulse to the excitatory/inhibitory centre in the brain in which there could be a pre-existing disorder. This would cause the peripheral arteries to constrict rather than dilate, increasing the blood pressure.

If a patient reports dizziness, headaches, nervousness or elevated blood pressure a few hours after the seeds are put into the ears, ask the person to remove them. At the next treatment, use body acupoints instead of ear points.

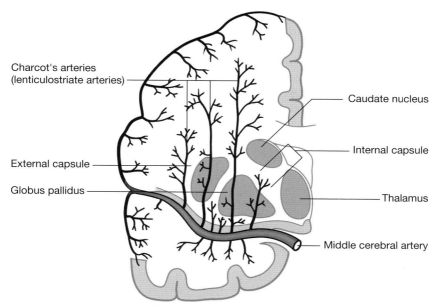

Figure 4.1 Arteries that branch off at right angles from the middle cerebral artery. These are particularly vulnerable to breakage when atherosclerosis or microaneurysm is present.

What to do in case of intracranial haemorrhage

During the treatment, if the patient develops headache, nausea, vomiting, weakness or confusion, don't wait until double vision, loss of speech, paralysis or unconsciousness develop before suspecting there is bleeding in the brain! Stop treatment immediately, remove all needles and check the patient's blood pressure while awaiting the ambulance. Ensure the patient is not moved until emergency medical assistance arrives.

It is all too easy to misjudge signs of brain haemorrhage as merely needle fainting, or hypoglycaemia that results in fainting during a strong treatment. In these less serious cases, a practitioner would commonly employ acupressure or acupuncture on Du-26, between the nose and upper lip, to bring the patient back to consciousness. However, if the patient's history leads you to suspect a haemorrhage, or the blood pressure reading is at all high, this technique is dangerous as it will raise the blood pressure further.

Prevention of intracranial haemorrhage

If a prospective patient comes in with high blood pressure, it is advisable not to give acupuncture unless the person has already seen a medical doctor and the blood pressure is reasonably under control with medication or other therapy. This is true whether the person is seeking acupuncture for the hypertension or for some other complaint. People with a history of blood pressure problems should also be given gentle treatments.

People who have had strokes often request acupuncture to alleviate common poststroke deficits such as paralysis, vision problems or speech impairments. The correct length of time to wait before beginning to treat a poststroke patient is still under discussion.

As a general guideline, it is important not to begin acupuncture treatment until all bleeding has stopped and the patient's blood pressure and general condition are completely stable. In Western countries, where acupuncturists do not commonly work in hospitals alongside physicians, the doctor's approval will be necessary. Even after the patient has returned home, it is a good idea to communicate with the physician before beginning poststroke acupuncture therapy.

Treatment should be extremely gentle to begin with; choose only a few points, keep stimulation gentle and increase the strength of treatment very gradually over a month or so, to allow the patient's body to adjust to it. For patients whose stroke is quite recent, it is preferable to avoid the use of sensitive points such as Du-20, Du-26, KI-1 or the 12 Well points. Excessive stimulation of qi too soon could trigger another stroke.

We know that certain points are bidirectional; in other words, the same points can be used to raise or lower blood pressure. The therapeutic effect of these points is entirely dependent on technique. Strong stimulation, which will raise blood pressure, may be dangerous to a stroke patient. Gentler stimulation will lower blood pressure. PC-6, SP-6 and ST-36 are recommended in many textbooks for their usefulness in regulating blood pressure in the desired direction (Ma 1992).

During treatment, observe the patient closely. If there are any warning signs of an impending stroke, such as headache, dizziness or confusion, cease treatment immediately, remove all needles and contact the emergency services.

In this section we have been talking about patients with haemorrhagic stroke. In the case of ischaemic stroke, which is more common, we can safely begin treatment sooner after the event to assist the patient's rehabilitation toward full function.

MENSTRUAL HAEMORRHAGE

When a woman comes for acupuncture treatment for conditions unrelated to her reproductive system, the practitioner may not be aware of whether or not she is menstruating at the time. If the patient is having her period, the use of certain points can inadvertently trigger menstrual flooding.

Case study 4.4

A 28-year-old woman sought acupuncture treatment for discomfort in her upper stomach, and a feeling of fatigue in her legs when she walked. Unbeknownst to the practitioner, the patient was on the 3rd day of her period. Points SP-6 and GB-34 were chosen. After the needles had been in for 15 minutes, the patient began to feel pain in her lower abdomen, especially in the areas of the ovaries and fallopian tubes. The practitioner removed all the needles. The cramping was so severe the woman was unable to lie down on her back; her lower abdomen was swollen, hard and painful. She went to the bathroom, where she began to have a heavy flow of dark-red blood with small clots. The flooding relieved the cramps, and after the woman had rested in the clinic for 20 minutes, she was feeling well enough to walk home. Four days later, she returned for examination, and reported all was well (Yang 1958).

So far, this is the only fully described case that has come up in the literature. The phenomenon is well known to experienced practitioners, however; it may be that because a single episode of menstrual flooding is not dangerous to the patient it tends not to be reported.

Related acupoints

LI-4
ST-25
SP-6
BL-23–BL-34, BL-40, BL-60, BL-67
GB-21
Ren-2 – Ren-7
Du-2 – Du-4

Discussion of menstrual haemorrhage

Normal menstruation – the shedding of the lining of the uterus, accompanied by some bleeding, at roughly monthly intervals – can easily be affected by acupuncture. The use of certain points, as well as the stimulation of acupuncture, which causes uterine contractions, may rupture small blood vessels. This may result in cramps and bleeding that is heavier than usual. When treating a woman of child-bearing age we should choose our points with caution if they have the potential to affect menstruation.

Of course, there are circumstances in which we do use SP-6, BL-23, BL-32 and Ren-3, among others, during a woman's period to open meridians and clear qi and blood stagnation. The main examples are in treatment of irregular menses, dysmenorrhoea, fibroids or endometriosis. But even when encouraging blood flow is our purpose, it is important to refrain from excessive stimulation. In general, unless there is a specific treatment objective, we want to avoid setting off uterine cramping and bleeding.

The related points listed here come from three sources: the obvious proximity of acupoints on the middle and lower back to the uterus, advice from ancient classical literature and finally from the results of experiments done by modern-day medical researchers.

One study was done at the TCM Research Institute of China, Zhejiang Medical University, where patients' uterine contractions were monitored as acupuncture was performed on SP-6. The researchers' graphs revealed that, regardless of whether needle stimulation is performed by hand or electrical pulse, the uterus can begin to contract after 15–20 minutes' retention of the needle, and contractions may continue until they reach a peak as much as 20 minutes after the needle is withdrawn. This study clearly shows that if SP-6 is stimulated during the patient's menstruation it is likely to increase flow and cramps (TCM Research Institute of Zhejiang Medical University 1973).

Although detailed studies have not been carried out on all points with a potential for inducing uterine contractions, some writers suggest that other points such as LI-3 may also have this effect. One of these papers lists a number of points that are contraindicated for use during menstruation, which are included in 'Related acupoints' above (Qicai 2000).

What to do in case of menstrual haemorrhage

If a woman undergoing acupuncture during her period suddenly starts to experience heavy cramps and significantly heavier bleeding, possibly accompanied by dizziness, lightheadedness, thirst, restlessness, sweats, palpitations and pallor, during or just after treatment, this is obviously a menstrual haemorrhage. Stop treatment and allow the patient to rest, using moxa on Du-8 and SP-1. You may also use herbs to reduce the bleeding. If the haemorrhage cannot quickly be brought under control with these measures, the patient may need to be sent for medical treatment. She may also need to take iron supplements to prevent or treat anaemia.

Prevention of menstrual haemorrhage

If a female patient of child-bearing age is complaining of hormonally related symptoms, such as heavy flow, premenstrual syndrome, etc., it is wise to inquire whether she is having her period at the time of treatment. If the woman is seeking help for an unrelated condition, but many of the points are in the abdominal area, ask about her cycle and avoid the points in the list. One example of this would be acupuncture for relief of insomnia; our common choice of SP-6 could aggravate menstrual bleeding, so an alternative point should be selected.

Even when a patient is expecting her period within a day or so, choose points other than those on the list, do a gentle treatment and observe the patient closely for signs of haemorrhage. Even if you avoid the most sensitive points and needle those just above and below it on the same meridian, the reaction of the energy flow through the meridian may still trigger bleeding. In TCM terminology this is known as a meridian bleeding reaction.

MISCARRIAGE RELATED TO ACUPUNCTURE

Related acupoints

LI-4
ST-12, ST-25
SP-6
BL-23 – BL-37, BL-60, BL-67
GB-21
LIV-1
Ren-2 – Ren-13
One or two references have also listed: LIV-3 and ST-36.

Please note that, although many of these points are the same as those associated with menstrual haemorrhage, a few such as LIV-1, ST-12 and some of the Ren points are not. This leads us to wonder what factors besides uterine contractions might be involved in a miscarriage, and how these may be influenced by acupuncture.

Discussion of miscarriage

Acupuncture is quite helpful in resolving the Spleen and Stomach qi deficiency or Liver–Stomach disharmony that cause pregnant women to suffer from morning sickness. Unlike some medications, acupuncture has no detrimental effects on the baby. However, the first trimester of pregnancy is the time when 85% of miscarriages occur. Usually a miscarriage in the first 12 weeks is the result of abnormality in the fetus, and would have occurred anyway regardless of whether the mother had had acupuncture or avoided it.

However, if there is risk of miscarriage because of some problems in the mother, acupuncture may in fact trigger this event if points that induce uterine contractions are used, or if stimulation is too strong. Once the pregnancy has reached its full term, needling of these points may be employed to stimulate smooth, effective contractions and reduce labour pain.

Because it is extremely difficult to determine one specific reason for a miscarriage early in pregnancy, the medical literature so far does not point to any definitive evidence of a cause-and-effect relationship between acupuncture and spontaneous abortion. Any reports are sprinkled with words like 'possibly' and 'maybe'. This is why there is no case study included here. However, several authoritative classical Chinese texts emphasise that certain points should not be used during pregnancy because of the risk of 'fetus dropping' or, in other words, miscarriage. Also, anecdotal reports from modern-day practitioners' clinical experience indicate that miscarriage happens often enough in conjunction with acupuncture, especially related to the points listed, to indicate the need for extreme caution. In most of these informal reports, either the practitioner is not aware that the woman is pregnant, or does not know that some commonly used points are risky.

If a patient loses her baby within a few weeks after acupuncture during which the practitioner has worked on sensitive points, can we prove the treatment caused the miscarriage? No. But there is enough evidence for a strong suspicion, and for avoiding this possibility by planning treatment properly.

Another factor that has not been fully explored in studies is the influence acupuncture has over the levels of hormones such as oestrogen and progesterone. Acupuncture is known to have profound effects, from centuries of experience in using this therapy to alleviate premenstrual syndrome and menopausal symptoms caused by hormonal fluctuations. And we know that oestrogen and progesterone levels change during pregnancy. Might acupuncture during pregnancy significantly affect the levels of these hormones enough to play a role in causing miscarriage? A good research study of this question would be a valuable addition to modern science's understanding of acupuncture.

What to do in case of miscarriage

It is likely, in a normal treatment, that if a patient has not informed the acupuncturist that she is pregnant and the practitioner has not thought to ask, the common points used will include some that are associated with risk of miscarriage. If, during the few days following treatment, the woman develops early signs of miscarriage such as spotting or cramps, the course of acupuncture treatments should cease immediately.

The patient should be advised to rest in bed and avoid any physical exertion or sexual intercourse. If the spotting doesn't stop within a couple of days, or it gets worse, the patient should see her doctor for an ultrasound and other tests to ascertain whether the fetus is still alive, and whether anything can be done to save the pregnancy.

Prevention of miscarriage

When seeing a woman of child-bearing age, even if she is being treated for a condition unrelated to her reproductive system, you are advised to inquire where she is in her menstrual cycle, if any of the acupoints you plan to use are those that are contraindicated during pregnancy.

Of course, when you collect a full history from a first-time patient, any previous miscarriages are a 'red flag' that should alert you to this risk. Unless you know for sure that a woman is not pregnant – for instance you know she is using reliable birth control or she has told you she has just finished a menstrual period – avoid using sensitive points.

If a woman has a history of miscarriage and is trying to conceive but it is too early to tell whether she is pregnant, a responsible practitioner will not perform acupuncture or any other energy-moving therapy on her. In Chinese medical theory, repeated miscarriages are seen as a result of Spleen/Kidney qi deficiency, qi/blood deficiency, yin deficiency with internal Heat, or some combination of these. It is all too easy to trigger a spontaneous abortion, even without external stimulation. The fetus can be 'shaken' by emotional upset, excessive exercise or many other factors.

Although a miscarriage after acupuncture may simply be a coincidence, for the protection of patient and practitioner it is best to avoid needling a woman who is at any risk of losing her baby. Once she has made it safely through the first sensitive months, the careful use of moxa or herbs will help consolidate the pregnancy and assist in developing a strong, healthy child.

When treating a woman who is having a normal pregnancy, in addition to avoiding use of the points listed above, during the first 3 months we refrain from using any abdominal points under the line of the umbilicus. After the first trimester, steer clear of all abdominal points, as the uterus is beginning to rise in the abdominal cavity. Back points, as we know, are connected to powerful meridians and may set off uterine contractions. Therefore all back points should be left alone throughout the entire pregnancy, except during labour itself, when their action will encourage productive contractions.

ACUPUNCTURE ACCIDENT PREVENTION STRATEGIES

As we have seen in the preceding sections, accidents in acupuncture are most commonly the result of incorrect angle or depth of needle insertion, or both. A correct angle is especially important. Injuries also occur when the practitioner is trying too aggressively to obtain de qi. Remember that de qi is not necessarily achieved by more depth, or by stronger stimulation.

The more acupuncturists keep in mind the possibility of an accident, the more careful they will be in technique, and therefore an accident is less likely to occur. Every time a practitioner is about to insert a needle, a few moments should be taken to consider whether the angle and depth are correct. It is better to verify questionable points until they are all committed to memory, rather than to guess. Textbooks give an average depth and angle for an average person. Few people fit the average profile! Adjusting needle insertions to match an individual's size and constitution becomes easier with experience.

For an acupuncturist, one of the most important accident prevention strategies is to keep the mind focused and the spirit peaceful. Personal concerns must be placed to the side while you concentrate on the job at hand. Here is a focusing exercise that may be helpful:

Focusing exercise

1. Take a deep breath.
2. State your intent to yourself, saying 'Right now I must focus on this treatment and anything else I will not worry about until this patient leaves.'
3. Focus your vision for several seconds on the tip of each needle before inserting it.
4. Visualise the acupoint on the skin as precisely as if you were actually drawing a ring around it; are there any blood vessels or nerves nearby that must be avoided? Is there any reason the use of this point might be inappropriate for this patient?

Another common error occurs when a needle bends underneath the skin and the practitioner manipulates it without sensing the bend (Fig. 4.2). The key here is to leave the needle alone after each thrust in order to observe its natural resting angle. This angle will change if the needle is bent (Fig. 4.3).

Carelessness with needles

One kind of carelessness is when the practitioner finishes the treatment but forgets to remove a needle from the patient's body. Another is when a needle

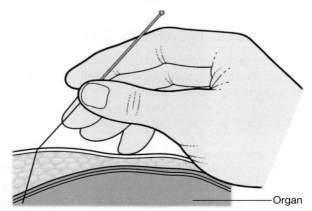

Organ

Figure 4.2 A bending needle. Many injuries are caused when the practitioner is unaware that the needle is bending, and continues to force it.

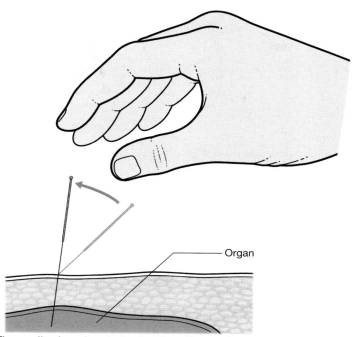

Figure 4.3 The needle gives clues to its direction. Observe the natural resting angle between thrusts.

falls out unseen, and is lost in the patient's clothing or belongings, or in the treatment bedding. These situations can cause accidents and may damage the reputation of your clinic or even result in legal problems.

Expose the treatment area thoroughly. Move collars, sleeves and other pieces of clothing well out of the way, or ask the patient to remove them. Trouser legs or sleeves can easily slide down and obscure a needle. Never cover needles with a blanket; it is possible to forget about them.

If a needle is left in the patient's arm or leg, the person is likely to feel a little pain when standing up or walking around. But if it is left in the hair it won't be felt, and can fall out later and cause an injury if stepped on. Some practitioners count the needles before and after treatment.

Another useful trick is to cut arrows about an inch or an inch and a half (2.5–3 cm) long from brightly coloured paper or plastic, and place them on the bed and pillow, pointing toward the needle locations (Fig. 4.4). These are eye-catching reminders of where the needles are placed. It also helps to use longer needles (1.5–2 cun) on points that are difficult to see, such as those on the top of the head, the back and side of the neck, and on the extremities where clothing may hide the needle.

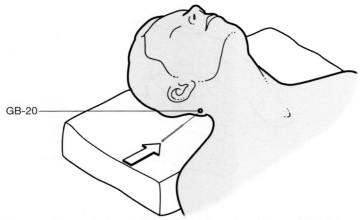

Figure 4.4 Eye-catching reminders of the location of needles that are difficult to see.

A 'stuck' needle is not, strictly speaking, the result of carelessness, although lack of care in withdrawal can injure the patient. Stuck needles are included in so many reports about adverse effects that the subject is worth a short review.

Every teacher will receive at least one phone call from students practising needling on each other, who are in a panic because the needle won't come out, or can't be moved when stimulation is attempted. Do not yank the needle out by force! The correct procedure is to place needles on the 'upper and lower storey' points above and below the stuck needle. Or a moxa stick can be circled around the stuck needle to warm and relax the tissues. After 2 or 3 minutes of either treatment, the needle will be released.

Broken needles are increasingly rare, as the use of disposable needles, which have not been weakened by repeated sterilisation, is mandatory in many countries and strongly urged in most others.

Carelessness with patients

Strange as it may seem, distracted acupuncturists have been known to forget about a patient lying in a treatment room. One woman who posted her story on the internet says that she was left unattended with needles in her for more than an hour, during which time she began to feel shaky and chilled.

When it became clear the acupuncturist was not coming back, the woman removed the needles herself and left the office. It is unlikely a patient would be a proponent of acupuncture after such an experience. Whether you treat only one person at a time or book overlapping appointments, it is crucial to check in on the patient every few minutes to make sure treatment is proceeding as planned and that the patient is feeling comfortable and free of pain, anxiety or any other unpleasant effects from beginning to end of the acupuncture process.

References

Hao Xinwu 1986 Manic outburst caused by acupuncture. Beijing TCM College Journal 6:29

Ma Zhongxue 1992 Acupuncture international exchange handbook. Shandong Science and Technology Publishing House, Jinan

Qicai W 2000 Prohibition of acupuncture during menstruation. International Journal of Clinical Acupuncture 11:319-320

TCM Research Institute of Zhejiang University, Hangzhou 1973 Needling some points can cause uterine contractions. Science & Technology Bulletin 6:1

Shi Yongxing 1987 Acupuncture and herb injection improve chronic primary low blood pressure. New TCM Journal (11):31

Yang Meiliang 1958 Three cases of acupuncture treatment causing abdominal cramps and hemorrhage during menstrual period. Shanghai TCM and Herb Journal 9:28

Zhou Tianqi et al 1985 Fatal intracranial hemorrhage caused by acupuncture: one case report. Xinjian TCM and Herb Journal 4:24

Accident prevention with other techniques

5

When a patient's condition does not seem to be improving in the time period we would expect, practitioners have a large toolbox of additional techniques to draw upon. Special techniques such as electrical stimulation, ear acupuncture, gua sha, etc. are of great benefit in many situations where acupuncture alone is not effective enough. This chapter supplements the basic instruction you have received in these techniques with more detailed information on the indications and precautions for each one.

ELECTRICAL STIMULATION

Of all the supplementary techniques, electroacupuncture is the most commonly used. But it is not appropriate for every patient. For many people, even the lowest intensity feels too strong, and inhibits relaxation.

We should be very careful when using electrical stimulation on patients suffering from mental and spiritual imbalances (such as depression and anxiety) because the extra intensity of the bioelectric pulse may aggravate the patient's agitation. The technique can be used successfully on people with schizophrenia or severe insomnia, but it is advisable to begin gently and observe these patients with extreme care during treatment.

Tolerance to the sensation of electricity is very individual. You should observe each individual patient's tolerance range and record it for future reference. An individual patient's tolerance may alter during the course of treatment. A weakening patient tends to become more sensitive. A patient who is overstimulated (i.e. intensity is too strong or duration too long) will, after treatment, feel soreness unrelated to the original complaint. Adjust intensity in small, slow increments and ask patients how they are tolerating the stimulation at each step.

The choice of correct waveform depends on the patient's complaint and the purpose of treatment. The dense wave relaxes muscles so it is best for pain. The disperse wave excites tissues so it is the waveform of choice for weakness. The dense-and-disperse wave setting promotes qi and blood circulation so it is best for reducing oedema, making it ideal in treatment of injuries and inflammation.

Precautions for electrical stimulation are important to remember because accidents can have serious repercussions. Avoid placing the electric leads in such a way that the current can pass through the heart or spinal cord, for instance on the left and right side of the chest, or on two points along the spinal cord. Electric stimulation can disrupt the cardioelectric field of the heart and nervous system, which may cause arrhythmia, fibrillation or cardiac arrest. The technique is contraindicated for people with cardiac pacemakers; the pulse of the electrical stimulator will override the pacemaker's rhythm. It is also best to avoid using electricity on pregnant women.

After each treatment, turn all dials to zero and check the dials on the apparatus again before treating the next patient. Some people have been jolted when they have been hooked up to an electrostimulator that was still on a high setting from a previous patient. This is not only uncomfortable but potentially dangerous.

It should be pointed out that electroacupuncture stimulators vary widely in quality. Some stimulators have been known to emit a high-frequency current that degrades the needle and causes tissue damage in the patient. An electrical stimulator should be able to be calibrated, and before use on patients should be tested to ensure that its frequencies and waveforms match the standards claimed in the manual.

As with acupuncture in general, sudden strong stimulation or too much electrical stimulation of some sensitive points can overexcite the parasympathetic nerves. One branch of the parasympathetic nerve fibre runs from the vagus nerve and controls part of the heart function. This means that a vagus reflex can create a disturbance of the cardioelectric field.

A few examples of this are found in the literature; in three separate cases, electrical stimulation of ST-6, LI-18 and Ex. An Mian triggered vagus reflexes that resulted in dropping blood pressure, heart arrhythmia and loss of consciousness in the patient. All cases recovered with CPR and drugs like atropine, which is a vagus antagonist.

A way to check ahead of time whether a patient has a very sensitive vagus nerve is to press slowly and carefully on the person's closed eyelids for 10 seconds with your thumbs or index fingers, and then check the pulse. If it has slowed to 10 beats/minute, the person has a sensitive vagus nerve and it would be advisable to choose distal points rather than those on the chest or the neck, to make the treatment gentler. Always find out whether patients have any history of arrhythmia or other heart condition, particularly if they are elderly.

The body needs to be given a chance to adapt gradually to electrical stimulation. Increase the level very slowly, remaining at each increment for 5 minutes. There is a case in China of a man with schizophrenia whose condition was being treated using electrical stimulation to points on the temple and neck. This set off a full-body spasm that was strong enough to fracture the neck of his femur.

Constant observation and communication are important. When treating a condition such as Bell's palsy, small, local muscle spasms are an acceptable, even desirable, effect of stimulation. But electric acupuncture must never be aggressive enough to cause large muscle spasms.

AURICULAR ACUPUNCTURE

Ear acupuncture is a commonly used supplementary technique because it is useful in so many situations. Auricular acupuncture may be done with regular needles, tacks, or ear seeds or metal beads. It works well on hyperactive primary school children, for attention deficit disorder, facial twitching and inability to concentrate.

It is a good treatment for almost everybody, and can be used preventatively for conditions such as eyestrain caused by excessive reading or computer use. Ear acupuncture is becoming popular worldwide in treatment of drug, alcohol and tobacco addictions either alone or in combination with regular body points. As it boosts metabolism and reduces hunger sensations, it is also an effective way to promote weight loss.

In ear acupuncture, the main concern is infection. Because of the current popularity of the technique of embedding needles, an increasing number of outer ear infections are being reported. There is little or no subcutaneous tissue between the skin and cartilage of the ear, and cartilage has no blood vessels. Where there is poor circulation, the body has no way to send immune cells to fight infection, which then spreads easily from the skin to the cartilage. If infection is not treated promptly and effectively, the cartilage may become permanently deformed.

The type of bacteria commonly implicated in such infections is *Pseudomonas*, which has an affinity for body parts such as ear cartilage. Of nine cases of acupuncture-related cartilage infection treated in a 7 year period at a hospital in Nanjing, six turned out to be *Pseudomonas* (Nanjing Drum Tower Hospital 1973).

If redness and swelling do occur, remove the needles and warm the affected area with a moxa stick one or two times a day for 15 minutes each time. Some herbs are helpful in clearing infection in the early stages. A list of these is found in the section on Needling infection in Chapter 3.

Hygiene is the best defence against infection. Sterilise the patient's ears with both iodine and alcohol. If previous treatment has left redness or swelling around a particular acupoint, avoid further treatment on that spot.

It is risky to let patients go home with ear tacks taped in place, especially during the warm months, because it is nearly impossible to ensure that they will keep the area dry during and after showering or perspiring heavily. More practitioners now use regular needles during the treatment and remove them, then place ear beads, which have only a tiny sticker that allows air to reach the surface.

Although the use of such tiny needles would seem to be quite safe, there are a few other cautions. Like body acupuncture and electrical stimulation, auricular acupuncture can cause needle fainting. The vagus reflex responsible for this, and information on prevention and treatment of fainting, is discussed in detail in the section on Needle fainting in Chapter 4. The vagus reflex also seems to be implicated in cases where patients were given ear seeds to treat high blood pressure. Although many of these treatments have been successful, sometimes the blood pressure has actually been raised instead of lowered. This unexpected effect is far less likely to occur with body acupuncture.

Some experts also suggest that needles should not be used on auricular points of pregnant women. Ear acupuncture often has a stronger effect than body acupuncture. If done during the first 12 weeks of pregnancy, it may cause miscarriage. In the 8th and 9th months, there is danger of starting labour prematurely. For women who are seeking help in, for instance, stopping smoking, and who are in their 5th to 7th month of pregnancy, ear beads or seeds are a safer alternative as they do not appear to stimulate uterine contractions. However, a pregnant patient should be closely watched during treatment. If a woman has any history of repeated miscarriage, even if she is just trying to conceive and it is not known whether she is pregnant, neither needles nor ear beads should be used.

PLUM BLOSSOM NEEDLE TECHNIQUE

Plum blossom needling is effective in encouraging the flow of qi and blood towards a problem area. It is useful in treating conditions such as eczema, psoriasis and alopecia, and numbness of the skin. However, this technique is less frequently used than others since the skin often shows red marks and sometimes wounds that look like cat scratches. These may last up to 5 days after treatment, and make patients feel uncomfortable with their appearance. As with cupping and gua sha, it is imperative to explain thoroughly to patients the possible visible after-effects, and find out whether they are comfortable with this.

Tapping strength varies according to each patient's sensitivity and the area of treatment. On the head and face it should be gentle; the skin remains unbroken. Medium-strength tapping elsewhere on the body causes darker redness but still no broken skin. Heavy technique resulting in tiny visible blood spots is indicated for severe vomiting, diarrhoea and lower back spasm.

As with any procedure that may break the skin, infection is a possibility. Before treatment clean the area with alcohol. If heavy tapping will be done, use iodine as well as alcohol. Disposable needle heads are best, or very strict sterilisation practices if you must reuse heads.

Finish a plum blossom treatment by cleaning the skin with a dry cotton ball, and advise the patient to keep the skin dry for several hours.

CUPPING

Cupping is a fairly common practice because it is quick, strong and effective. Its temporary visible after-effects can lead to misunderstanding, however, especially in countries where most people are unfamiliar with Chinese medicine. I once received a phone call from a local police officer who was inquiring about the round bruises a teacher had reported seeing on an Asian boy's neck and back. The child's mother had given him a cupping treatment. I reassured the police officer that it was not abuse and faxed him information about the technique.

Be aware that there can be too much of a good thing in this kind of treatment. One acupuncturist in Australia used more than 70 cups at a time on a single patient, resulting in blistering and reddening over most of the person's back. The concern here is not merely painful blistering or burns. Excessive cupping can cause soft tissue damage so severe that its chemical composition changes, releasing dead cells and toxicity into the bloodstream.

This overload can lead to kidney failure. It is much like 'crush syndrome' from a fall or from being buried in earthquake debris. While a patient with chronic severe back pain may require treatment with 10 to 12 cups at a time, there is never any need to go beyond this limit.

Do not use cupping at all on patients with cancer, heart conditions, haemophilia or severe oedema.

Careful technique will prevent injury. Take care not to overheat the cup edge and burn the patient's skin. Heat the air, not the cup, by holding it with the opening upwards and quickly circling the flame inside the jar. If the flame or an alcohol drop touches the edge, dry it and heat a second time.

After cupping, there will sometimes be a blister of lymphatic fluid on the patient's skin. This is a breeding ground for infection, so if you see a blister it is important to take preventive action. Use 70% alcohol to clean the skin on and around the blister. Then take a thick acupuncture needle and puncture the skin near the base of the blister, on all four sides, to allow the fluid to drain (Fig. 5.1). After that, dry the skin with a clean cotton ball. Once the blister has deflated, dress it with a gauze bandage soaked in alcohol and bandage it firmly to keep the skin from tearing. A day or two later, the skin should have adhered to the flesh again.

Figure 5.1 Draining lymphatic fluid from a blister to speed healing.

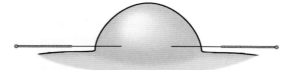

It is also important to clean cups thoroughly with alcohol after each treatment, to avoid transmitting contamination from lymphatic fluid and blood to the next patient. Cups may also be washed with soap and water first, then with iodine and alcohol, especially if you see any blood on them.

If you are doing bleeding cupping, it is probably better to discard the cups after the treatment; the patient may be charged accordingly to cover the extra expense.

GUA SHA

Gua sha is a valuable home remedy, like massage, which can be taught to patients, although its therapeutic benefits are often stronger. It involves scraping the skin of the back from the neck to the lower back until redness appears. As its technique is not generally taught in English language texts, it is included here.

Gua sha is similar to cupping in that it must be described carefully to the patient, in order to prepare the person for the resulting temporary changes to the appearance of the skin. Although a spoon, coin or comb may be used, the preferred tool is a thick rounded-edged soupspoon. The edge of the tool should not be sharp.

Gua sha is good at releasing toxins and pathogenic factors from the body's surface, so it is indicated for fever, headache and body aches due to severe colds and flu, food poisoning or sunstroke.

Start from the medial lines Du meridian and work outward. In most cases the practitioner would work on only three lines (Du and the two middle

Bladder meridians); in a more serious case of flu one might add the Ex. Hua Tuo Jia Ji lines for a total of five (Fig. 5.2). The use of all seven lines is rare, and is indicated only at the peak of a severe cold or influenza, when the patient has chills and fever, and only if the patient has a strong enough constitution to tolerate it.

The back should first be lubricated with 70% alcohol, vegetable oil or massage oil. Scrape in one direction only, along each meridian, from the base of the neck to the lower back with long, even strokes, 20 times on each line. Afterwards wipe the lubricant off the skin with a clean cloth and cover the person with a blanket to rest. Advise the patient not to eat cold or greasy food for a few days.

A strong treatment may break the skin slightly, allowing minute quantities of red blood cells to leak out. Because of the overall redness in the skin, this tiny amount of bleeding will be nearly invisible to the practitioner. But, as American acupuncturist and educator David C. Kailin (1997) points out, it is still enough to pose a risk of transmission of viruses such as hepatitis B and HIV. This is also a potential hazard with cupping.

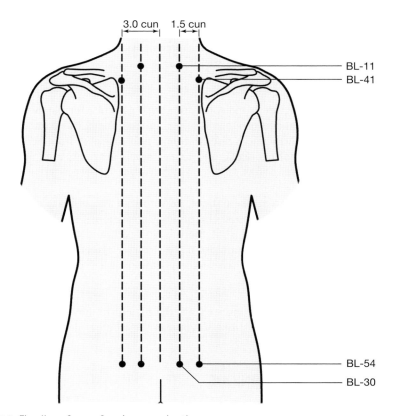

Figure 5.2 Five lines for performing gua sha therapy.

To ensure that no blood and toxins are transferred from one patient to the next, it is important to clean the scraper thoroughly with soap and water, iodine, then alcohol and dry it thoroughly before and after each treatment. Kailin's view is that the scraping tool should be something that is single use and disposable.

SCALP ACUPUNCTURE

Scalp acupuncture elicits a strong reaction in about half the patients who experience it – a heavy achy feeling throughout the body that is often uncomfortable after the treatment. Therefore, when you decide to try this technique, do it gently with only one or two needles and find out how your patient responds to it. It is important to proceed with caution and to develop trust with your patient.

The scalp is rich in blood vessels, so it is necessary to use a large cotton ball and to press points for longer than usual after withdrawing the needles to stop any bleeding. In order to maintain clean needle technique, use the fingers of your other hand to keep the patient's hair away from the needle as it is being inserted.

Scalp tissue is tight so the needle sensation is often strong; watch for needle fainting. Check to see how the patient is feeling during the treatment; afterward ask the person to sit in your waiting area for at least 5 minutes before going home.

Scalp acupuncture is indicated for stroke patients, for paralysis following cerebral haemorrhage or embolism, for aphasia and facial paralysis, and for Parkinson's and Alzheimer's disease. It may also ease pain from nerve disorders such as trigeminal neuralgia, and relieve severe dizziness and tinnitus from inner ear disorders.

When treating a stroke patient, be sure that the primary care physician has been consulted to ensure the person's condition is stable, that all internal bleeding has stopped, that there is no fever, and that the heart is not weak. Because scalp acupuncture has a stronger effect than body acupuncture, there is an increased risk of complications if it is done too soon after a stroke.

While the needles are inserted, ask the patient to move his or her body on the side affected by the stroke so you can see whether de qi has reached the affected limbs.

EMBEDDED NEEDLE TECHNIQUE

This is a technique practised in some countries in which a short needle or tack is implanted and retained in the patient's body for several days or even longer to extend the effective treatment period. It is used to treat severe neuralgia or chronic neurological conditions such as paralysis.

There are many reports of injury associated with this technique; in these cases the needle has migrated through the body and damaged tissue or, more seriously, the spinal cord, the heart, stomach or urinary bladder. Sheffield University Consultant Medical Acupuncturist Palle Rosted, MD describes a number of these in his online article 'Adverse reactions after acupuncture: a review' (2004).

The severity of such accidents has created an erroneous belief in the medical and general communities that acupuncture is dangerous. But most of the adverse effects cited in the literature are in fact associated with the improper use of embedded needles, or broken needles. The risk of infection is also high with this technique.

Many authorities no longer recommend the use of embedded needles, especially if a regular needle is cut up and used instead of one with a 'head' or bead at the top end. If special circumstances warrant the use of embedded needles, use the following safety precautions:

Safety precautions for using embedded needles

- Use only needles that have a bead at the end, to anchor them at the skin and prevent them from working their way into the body.
- Check the needles every day to make sure they have not moved, and that there are no signs of infection.
- Instruct the patient to keep the area clean and dry.
- If you must prolong the treatment, do not leave the same needles in for weeks. Give the patient a couple of days with no needles, then use fresh ones.

MOXA

Obviously, moxa cones and cigars can both cause burns if the practitioner is not careful. In a couple of reported cases, the patient suffered third degree burns. Our main concern here is to prevent further problems if a burn does occur; an infection of the site will cause more serious scarring than the burn itself. First aid for burns is covered in the section on Cupping.

There have been a few reports in the literature of patients fainting during moxa treatment. In these cases, the patient was already very weak from diarrhoea or heavy uterine bleeding. If you are seeing a patient who is in a weakened condition, don't assume that moxa is perfectly safe. A gentle or short treatment may be more appropriate. Watch for early signs of fainting.

Information on how to deal with this situation is found in the section on Needle fainting in Chapter 4.

TDP LAMP

This therapeutic lamp is now popular in many countries. It is included here because it has an interesting history, and because it has some specific safety issues associated with it.

This device was invented by a Dr Gou Wen Bin, who was an engineer at an enamel factory in Chongqing, China, which just happens to be my home town. Every spring, influenza tore through the city's workplaces and schools. Dr Gou started to wonder why, when so many employees of the Chongqing Enamel Factory were off sick with the flu, the ones in the coating and acid pickling department were still at work and seemingly fending off the virus. Obviously there was something being emitted from the enamelling process that appeared to bolster people's immune systems.

On further investigation, Dr Gou began to discover that the mysterious force wasn't a substance but an electromagnetic wave that was being absorbed by people's bodies. He performed many experiments using different materials from enamel coatings containing hundreds of combinations of trace elements, using electric heat on different materials. He found that when electricity was used to heat certain materials, these would radiate a part of the electromagnetic spectrum that could be absorbed by the human body. In 1979 he invented his lamp and did studies on lab mice and farm livestock. In experiments on seedlings, plants treated with the device were more resistant to disease and weather changes than were the control plants.

In 1981–2 I joined a research team that conducted clinical studies of the lamp on patients who had undergone abdominal surgeries such as appendectomy and hernia repair. We found that surgical sites treated with this lamp healed much faster than usual, with a lower rate of infection and minimal scar tissue.

TDP, when translated from the Chinese language, stands for Specific Electromagnetic Spectrum Device. It is often referred to, incorrectly, as a 'far-infrared radiator' or an 'ultrasonic therapeutic device'. Actually the lamp emits a large range of electromagnetic energy from 0.2 micrometres (ultraviolet) to at least 25 micrometres (infrared). There is no radioactivity. Its effects don't come from heat; heat is only the vehicle by which the wave is transmitted to the needles, making them vibrate at almost a microscopic level. The lamp's radiant ceramic plate contains more than 32 trace elements, which affect the kind of energy that is being radiated and also the biochemical functions of tissue.

For instance, oedema from lower back injury will be more quickly relieved (by 20–30%) with this therapy. It is also indicated for treating sports injuries, arthritis, dysmenorrhoea, irritable bowel and many other conditions. As it is much like an electronic form of moxa, it can be used on ST-36 of cancer patients to increase immune energy.

Contraindications include pregnancy; we don't yet know what if any effects this energy has on a fetus. Avoid using it close to the eyes; in theory it could contribute to development of cataracts. If the lamp is being used to treat acne, shield the patient's eyes. There is not yet enough research on the possible effect on the brain, so it is best not to aim it directly at the scalp. It should not be used directly on tumours, especially those of the breast, ovaries, uterus, lung and intestine. However, after a tumour has been surgically removed, there are some circumstances in which the lamp can be used therapeutically and safely, for instance when a postsurgical colon cancer patient is experiencing the effects of intestines narrowed by scar tissue.

Unfortunately, lots of accidents occur with this device because practitioners put the lamp over the patient's skin and walk away to do something else; 10 minutes later the patient can have suffered serious burns. Burns can of course occur when the lamp head is too close to the skin, but if it is too far away, there will be no therapeutic effect. The head should be placed, on average, 30 cm from the skin surface, but should be adjusted depending on whether the patient has tough or delicate skin. The treatment should result in an increase in skin temperature to no more than 40–42°C, only a few degrees higher than normal body temperature.

For children, seniors and others with sensitive skin, increase the distance. The correct distance also depends on which area of body is being treated. The head can be slightly closer when treating ankle and knee joints, but the tissue around the stomach and neck is thinner, so the lamp must be further away.

A 30 minute session with the heat lamp is enough for each treatment, as the increase in energy movement can make the patient feel lightheaded. Be aware that it takes 5–8 minutes for the ceramic head to preheat; practitioners sometimes assume it is not hot enough and place it too close to the patient's skin. In 10 minutes it will be hot enough to burn. It is imperative to check the heat and adjust the distance 8 or 9 minutes after putting on the device. The patient should not be left unattended.

Also, when buying these devices, be careful to check that the voltage is correct for use in your country. The quality of TDP lamps varies widely, so do some research to ensure you are buying a good-quality apparatus from a reputable company. The best clue is the presence of good insulation between the plate and the rest of the lamp head. Price is not necessarily an indication of quality.

Theoretically, the manufacturers say, the plates are good for 1000 hours. But who's counting? Here's a way to tell whether the plate needs replacement:

when it is new, it is black or at least a very dark grey; by the time it has become a mottled greyish white, it has lost its therapeutic value.

POST-TREATMENT SAFETY

Some treatments will leave a patient feeling extremely tired or debilitated. Most commonly this would happen after acupuncture, but it has been known to occur after a strong moxa, cupping or scalp acupuncture treatment. Patients may be so 'out of it' that they appear to be intoxicated. If you observe such a reaction in your patient, suggest that the person rests in your waiting area for 10 minutes or so, or perhaps takes a short walk before attempting to drive home. Driving long distances immediately after acupuncture is not a good idea; you may wish to caution your patient about this if you see the treatment has strongly affected the level of alertness.

References

Kailin DC 1997 Acupuncture risk management; the essential practice standards and regulatory compliance reference. CMS Press, Corvallis, Oregon

Nanjing Drum Tower Hospital 1973 Suppurative perichondritis of auricle caused by ear acupuncture. New Medicine Journal 7:339

Rosted P 2004 Adverse reactions after acupuncture: a review no. 2. Online. Available: http://users.med.auth.gr/~karanik/english/articles/adverse1.html

Ethics and interpersonal skills

INTRODUCTION

One of the fundamental tenets of Chinese medicine is the idea that the practitioner is treating a whole person, whose body, mind and spirit are inseparable, and who is intimately connected to, and influenced by, internal and external environment. When a person is asking for help with a health problem, part of this patient's environment is the practitioner. Thus, the question of whether it is preferable to see a medical professional who is a skilled diagnostician and technician or one who is an approachable and supportive healer shouldn't even arise in our discipline. A good TCM practitioner must be all of these things, and more.

Of course it is important for the acupuncturist to move beyond basic competence to ever-increasing levels of technical skill. But the intangible elements of the healing relationship are just as crucial to the success of treatment.

These intangibles include an attitude of acceptance and respect for others, a well-developed understanding of ethics and boundaries and an ability to truly listen to people and comprehend their needs, whether or not these are expressed verbally.

They also include practitioners' emotional maturity and stability, self-confidence without excessive ego, and an ongoing effort to nurture and develop their own healing qi, to assist patients' recovery without draining their own reserves. All encounters with patients involve an exchange of physical, mental and emotional energy, and it is up to practitioners to ensure that this energy is as clean, clear and healthy as possible.

This section introduces the Tao of the healing relationship, in the hope that it will encourage readers to explore these ideas in more depth and enrich their practice.

Ethical issues in acupuncture practice

6

Ethics is a branch of philosophy that concerns values relating to human conduct, and whether actions and the motivations for these actions are right or wrong. In traditional Chinese culture, ethical behaviour is expressed in the Tao. As Lao Tzu's *The Tao of Power, the Classic Guide to Leadership, Influence and Excellence* puts it: 'The Tao produces, its moral power supports; its natural law forms; its influence completes'.

As acupuncturists, we have responsibilities to our patients, the general public, other health care practitioners and to ourselves. Although it would take an entire book to cover the subject in depth, and in fact there are many books on medical ethics, a selection of basic ethical issues is explored here because the subject is rarely given more than a brief mention in most schools of Chinese medicine.

Acupuncturists are faced with many ethical decisions in their day-to-day practice. The purpose of this section is to help individuals develop standards that ensure patient safety and rights and practitioners' own legal protection, without necessarily abandoning the traditional philosophies of healing that make acupuncture and TCM special.

Ethics in TCM are rooted in the philosophies of Taoism, Buddhism and Confucianism. Each has had its own particular influence. Confucius promoted social stability and a sense of duty to society, which eventually found their way into the principles of treating individual people. Saving a person's life is the same idea as saving the world. A Confucian doctor cultivates a high degree of moral character, thinks through all the consequences before proceeding with treatment and treats patients with the care and loyalty he would give to his country. Confucianism is the relationship between the human being and society.

Taoism on the other hand is based on the relationship between a human being and nature. Although Taoism as a philosophy and spiritual practice began much earlier than the time of Confucius, its principles became more widespread in medical thinking at around the same time. But as the feudal power structures found Confucianism useful to its own ends, Taoism became somewhat marginalised.

Taoists have always had less of a connection with the power structures and have been more involved with the poor and working classes. They seek immortality, and therefore put much effort into health practices such as exercise and the development of medications, such as immortality pills. They created an advanced system of herbology and technical innovations such as acupuncture, which, even if they didn't quite make people live forever, certainly improved health and longevity.

The guiding principle of Taoist medicine is to restore harmony between the human body and the energies of nature, not only to cure but also to prevent disease. Taoists also believe that saving people from death and suffering helps the physician accumulate virtue, which contributes to his or her own spiritual immortality.

Buddhism has greatly influenced the development of TCM ethics. Its precepts list a number of things that a Buddhist medical practitioner should not do. These include not taking the life of a sentient being, not charging unreasonable fees and not practising under the influence of alcohol. A practitioner should also take the pain of others as his or her own, and help them to suffer less. Buddhist teachings help people climb out of the 'bitter ocean' that is the daily pain of existence, to respect life, develop compassion for others and cultivate an indifference to fame and wealth.

This is not to say one must be an adherent of an Eastern religion to be a good TCM doctor. But it does remind us that the basic principles of these traditions are still at the heart of the way we treat our patients and our own personal and professional behaviour – in other words, a framework for ethics. It is interesting to note how little some of the issues in human interaction have changed over thousands of years.

A historical perspective of ethical practice

Xia Cheng TCMD, MD (China), PhD, RAc

The development of ethics in Chinese medicine goes back thousands of years, and is revealed in the many stories of outstanding doctors and the principles that guided their work as healers.

The very first TCM doctor to be immortalised in the historical literature was Bian Que, a legendary half-man, half-god who practised as a physician, paediatrician and gynaecologist around 500BC. Dr Bian Que, who was also a famous acupuncturist, was not only skilled at pulse diagnosis but also had a special ability to detect illnesses in the internal organs. After he used acupuncture, moxibustion and hot herbal compresses to revive a prince of Guo, who had been declared dead and was about to be buried, stories spread that Bian Que could bring deceased people back to life. But this ethical doctor refused to be labelled a miracle-worker, saying that in truth the prince had not really been dead in the first place.

During the following few centuries, generations of doctors who lived and worked between 200BC and AD200 contributed their knowledge and ethics to the book that laid down the foundations of traditional Chinese medicine: the Huang Di Nei Jing, known in English as the *Yellow Emperor's Internal Classic*. This book differentiates between a Shang Gong – a doctor with superior skills – and a Cu Gong – one with lesser abilities. For example, in performing acupuncture, a Shang Gong knows how to give treatment based on the shen (spirit), but a Cu Gong can base treatments only on the patient's physical condition. During needling, a Shang Gong observes the qi coming and going, but a Cu Gong observes only physical points. A Cu Gong can also make mistakes, so that the original illness remains and a new illness starts from incorrect practice. The *Yellow Emperor's Internal Classic* emphasises that good skills in diagnosis and treatment are necessary to be a Shang Gong or superior doctor.

The pioneer of TCM's differentiation of syndromes was Dr Zhongjing Zhang (AD 150–219), who wrote the book Shang Han Za Bing Lun (*Treatise of Febrile and Miscellaneous Diseases*). The book's preface mentions that Dr Zhang always strove to learn from ancient and modern healers and to broaden his knowledge of medicine continuously from a wide range of sources. He also criticised careless doctors who wouldn't take time to collect enough detailed information from patients to be able to give an accurate diagnosis. Dr Zhang's commitment to continuing education and skill development has been a profound model for all TCM doctors who have come after him.

Knowledge and skill are one facet of ethics in Chinese medicine; equally important is the aspect of practising in the spirit of benevolence and altruism. This has been revealed in many stories of outstanding doctors and the principles that guided their work as healers.

One of these is Dr Dong Feng, who lived on Lushan Mountain, Jiangxi province during the Three Kingdoms Period (AD220–280). Dong Feng never refused patients no matter how ill they were. And he never received money for his services. Instead, he asked his recovered patients to thank him by planting apricot trees in his garden. Those who had been slightly ill were asked to plant one tree, those who had been seriously ill were asked to plant five. Years later, Dong Feng's garden had grown into an apricot orchard. In early spring, the trees blossomed. And in summer, the trees were overburdened with fruit. Every year when the apricots were ripe, Dong put a container in his granary and a notice on the wall, saying those who wanted to buy apricots could exchange grain for them. One container of apricots was worth one container of grain. People were trusted to do the exchange themselves without telling him. Dong kept a small quantity of grain for himself and gave the rest to poor orphans, widows, childless elderly people and travelers too hurried to have brought food with them. People spoke highly of Dong's kindness and manners.

His story has inspired generation after generation of TCM doctors to believe that the spirit of medical practice is to help people. In fact, Xinglin – which translates into 'forest of apricot trees' – became a word that means doctors.

The earliest article about TCM ethics was written by doctor Sun Simiao, who lived during the Tang Dynasty (AD618–907). This article, titled 'Da Yi Jing Cheng', which means 'great doctor', sets out the principles of a good practitioner.

First, a doctor has to be knowledgeable and highly skilled, and dedicated to continuously improving these skills to best serve the patients. Secondly, the doctor must have a professional manner, including positive attitudes, a serious demeanour, be properly dressed, confident and well grounded. He or she should also have a calm and harmonious spirit and mind, a sympathetic heart, a willingness to save people from suffering and be prepared to sacrifice his or her own interests – or even life – to save others.

A great doctor treats all people with equal kindness, whether they are rich or poor, old or young, male or female, friends or enemies, pretty or ugly. He or she is ready to help patients whether the case is difficult or easy, whether it is day or night, hot or cold, and regardless of the practitioner's own hunger, thirst or fatigue.

Dr Sun's list of things a doctor must *not* do includes: talking loudly, making flattering comments, gossiping, saying bad things about other doctors, focusing on making a profit from helping people, and prescribing expensive, difficult-to-find medicines to patients who are rich. Dr Sun Simiao was called

Yao Wang ('king of herbal medicine') because of his contribution to Chinese medicine.

In TCM, humanity and altruism are the heart of ethics. That is why the names of many Chinese pharmacies and clinics to this day include the word 'ren', which means benevolence and kindheartedness.

Although many of the basic principles developed by the earliest Chinese doctors remain relevant to modern-day acupuncturists, the environment in which most of us work has become far more complex in the past millennium or so. This is especially true where Chinese medicine is finding its way into other cultures that have different ways of thinking about health care, which presents a whole new set of ethical challenges.

The acupuncturist in the West: professional and ethical issues

Christopher Lam BSc, MD

Above and beyond the basic requirements in training, 'credentialling' and licensing for the acupuncturist there are, as with any other health care provider, important issues related to the practice of the profession and code of conduct. The acupuncturist needs to observe the same code of ethics that befits all health care providers. That includes acting in the patients' best interests, upholding confidentiality and patient autonomy, and providing the basic information that allows informed consent (Lo 1998). For the acupuncturist in a Western society there are also some special considerations. Although acupuncture, as an alternative or complementary therapy, is increasingly used in the West, its acceptance by the conventional medical community remains problematic (NIH Consensus Development Panel on Acupuncture 1998). Despite the emergence of acceptable research findings and studies on acupuncture therapy, its 'mechanism of action' remains elusive (Kaptchuk 2002). Traditional Chinese medical theories – including those of qi (vital energy), yin–yang polarity, Five Phases (or 'Elements'), channels or meridians, zang–fu (organ systems), and the Spirits – have few, if any, correlates in Western medicine. For instance, the Spleen in Chinese medicine denotes an organ *system* with its corresponding functional and energetic system, not just the organ of the spleen per se. The principles and theories of traditional Chinese medicine belong to a paradigm that is entirely different from that of Western biomedicine.

Despite discrepancies between the two medical systems, increasingly more Westerners have begun to accept Chinese medicine and acupuncture in part, or mainly, because of the philosophy behind it. Here 'philosophy' means the concept of holism, body–mind–spirit harmony, self-care, health promotion and maintenance, and preventive health care. Chinese medicine is implicitly patient oriented (as opposed to disease oriented). For these reasons, in addition to its empirical efficacy, Chinese health care – acupuncture, herbology, qigong, taiji and so on – has made significant inroads into Western society.

The increased acceptance of acupuncture notwithstanding, the practitioner has to be able to communicate in terms that the patient can understand. The acupuncturist's impression of the patient's syndrome pattern and remedy need to be put into layman's terms that make sense, without confusing or worrying the patient (again, the Spleen system in Chinese medicine pertains to, among other things, digestive functions – a far cry from the mere organ by the same name). Interestingly, this might not be any more difficult than it is for a medical doctor to explain to patients the pathophysiology and treatments for many diseases and, particularly, the modes of action of numerous Western drugs. In the West, biomedicine is the politically dominant medical system, and patients tend to take a great deal for granted. For example, they may not ask how Prozac really works (no one really knows), but will probably inquire as to exactly how herbs or acupuncture can help their mood disorder. The acupuncturist has to be ready for that. Nowadays accessibility to a great deal of information has enabled the public to become much more knowledgeable. This should facilitate, not hinder, the ability of the practitioner to discuss the conditions and therapies with patients.

Another aspect of communication is that between different health practitioners. There remain many artificial barriers between the disciplines. For the average Western physician, the concepts and terminology used by the acupuncturist may sound so foreign that they may be dismissed outright as archaic and 'unscientific'. There may also be fear of the unknown and a perception of competition for the same patients. On the other hand, the acupuncturist might feel intimidated by the Western doctor, who might be perceived – sometimes justifiably – as arrogant. Arrogance can be found in any discipline.

For the patient it is disconcerting or downright detrimental to be subjected to conflicting views from different health practitioners, especially when one practitioner negates the opinions and treatments of another, without the appropriate knowledge and communication between the practitioners. A good dose of humility is in order. Western physicians who know nothing about Chinese medicine or acupuncture ought not to disparage them. Acupuncturists not trained in Western medicine cannot ethically, from their position of authority, advise about biomedicine's treatments and drugs. Should acupuncturists discover a new pathology in the patient that is beyond their scope of knowledge or practice, they should not hesitate to contact the patient's family physician. If practitioners from different disciplines can communicate with patients (in layman's terms), can they not do so between themselves? Interprofessional barriers have no place when they put the patient's health at risk.

Possible adverse effects of complementary therapies, such as herb–drug incompatibilities or interactions, possible delays in diagnosis or in obtaining the most effective treatments for serious medical conditions, can largely be obviated with the proper exchange of information. Once the medical doctor gains trust, then appropriate referrals could be made to the acupuncturist. Building bridges between professionals is far more desirable than having barriers. All too often family doctors are unaware of their patients' consultations with and treatments by other health practitioners, and patient care becomes fragmented. Interprofessional respect, cooperation and collaboration can only enhance patient care and ensure continuity of care.

No one has a monopoly on the truth. All practitioners need to know their own strengths and limitations, as well as those of their therapeutic modalities. Practitioners need to consult with and learn from each other. Indeed it should be a challenge – and a rewarding endeavour – to compare notes and see where the paradigms differ or overlap, and how they might in practice complement one another.

Each practitioner needs to ensure that the therapeutic modality practised is efficacious, safe (Macpherson et al 2001) and affordable. There should be no exaggerated claims of 'cures' for myriad diseases, as are present in some less-than-discreet advertisements. (The acupuncture needles do not 'cure' as much as induce natural healing processes.) The patient must not be taken advantage of in any way. In other words, the practitioner ought to act with honesty, integrity and responsibility, putting the patient's interests first and avoiding conflicts of interest. These principles are fundamental to a professional; without them there can be no respect, trust and confidence.

Although it is important to keep up to date (what is there to stop the knowledgeable practitioner from mentioning endorphins, peptides, qi and shen in the same breath?), one would do well to recollect the foundation and philosophical influences – the history and tradition – of Chinese medicine. Taoism, Confucianism and Buddhism are major influences on Chinese society and health care. The perennial concepts of harmony with nature, harmony in human relationships, altruism, compassion and loving-kindness are central to these timeless philosophies, as they are to the holistic practice of Chinese medicine. The ethics of caring (Branch 2000) – a Western concept closely related to the Eastern ideals – should be the guiding principle of all practitioners. Out of that arises the need to attain proficiency, competence, skills, continuing education and professional development.

Western and Chinese medicine can work well together, often in a synergistic manner. A contemporary model of such integrated health care already exists in China. For patients, especially those with complicated and chronic illnesses, a multidisciplinary and integrated approach is optimal. Solid rapport with the patient, intent to act in the patient's best interests and, not least, compassion must be present. From that viewpoint, ethical behaviour for all health care practitioners would be one and the same.

LEGAL AND ETHICAL STANDARDS   *Hong Zhen Zhu*

Codes of ethics in acupuncture

In China, standards of acupuncture practice have not been codified in law. Instead they have arisen organically in the culture and individual practice over a couple of thousand years. Traditionally, patients have an understanding of TCM and trust in the healer's judgement, so they are more likely to accept mild adverse reactions from treatment without assuming malpractice on the part of the practitioner. However, this is changing in China as the practice of TCM is being influenced by standards of Western medical treatment, and as a result more formal codes of practice are developing.

In Europe, the UK, North America and elsewhere, acupuncture and other forms of TCM are also evolving. More and more jurisdictions are developing codes and standards of practice for acupuncturists. Some of these are national; other countries have regulatory bodies in some provinces or regions but not all. Information on where to find a few of the major ones is given in a 'Further reading' section at the end of this chapter.

All professions in the health care field have a well-developed code of ethics. Of course, many ethical concerns are common to all forms of health care. But acupuncture brings up some specific issues mainly because it is relatively new in many countries, so few members of the public or even other health care professionals are knowledgeable about what constitutes acceptable or unacceptable practices. Also, because there are so many different levels of recognition of this discipline in different parts of the world, in society at large as well as in formal codes, the onus is even more firmly on the part of each individual acupuncturist to develop and maintain the highest standards of ethical practice and behaviour.

Ethical standards common to health-related professions include:

- putting patients' interest first
- safety
- hygiene
- honesty
- integrity
- responsibility
- equality (no discrimination based on race, gender, etc.)
- respect for patients' privacy (in treatment, with records and in communicating with others)
- respect for other health care providers' knowledge and skills.

Ethical standards specific to TCM and acupuncture include:

- providing information and education on course of treatment and TCM
- encouraging self-responsibility for health and connecting patients with the self-healing power of nature

- teaching patients about illness prevention (rather than depending on curing disease)
- treating the root cause of disease rather than merely suppressing symptoms
- continuing to update education and skills in TCM and knowledge of modern science
- referral to another practitioner/health care provider if no improvement is seen after the course of treatment
- ensuring that training is sufficient when using techniques other than acupuncture (e.g. ear acupuncture, scalp acupuncture)
- ensuring use of special techniques or treatments (e.g. administering injections of herbs) is legally permitted
- employing clean needle technique (one-time use of disposable needles only).

Incompetence and malpractice in acupuncture

Malpractice, in the field of health care, is defined as the improper or negligent treatment of a patient. Allegations of malpractice may arise from the practitioner's insufficient anatomical knowledge or incompetent technique that leads to a patient's injury or death, failing to follow hygienic procedures, practising while impaired by alcohol, drugs or illness, or performing procedures not allowed within the scope of practice. It is within an acupuncturist's scope of practice to make a TCM diagnosis and to give advice on nutrition, taiji and Chinese herbs, but it is beyond this scope to make a medical diagnosis or to discuss medications with patients. In non-Asian countries, acupuncturists are usually not considered primary care providers, though this is changing in some jurisdictions.

In order to maintain the highest level of ethics, it is our responsibility to educate ourselves as much as possible by continuing to upgrade our own skills and knowledge, as well as reading medical journals and learning from practitioners in other disciplines.

Students and novice practitioners are often surprised and sometimes resentful when they are expected to know a certain amount of anatomy and biochemistry along with TCM theory and technique. Although our approach to healing is different from that of Western medicine, we still must respect and follow many rules of modern science. One example is in the use of sterile techniques. Bacteria don't refrain from attacking a patient's body just because the practitioner is using acupuncture needles instead of a scalpel.

In addition, patients often arrive with a Western medical diagnosis. They don't know the Chinese medicine category for their problem. If the acupuncturist does not fully understand what the patient's diagnosis means and what pathogenic changes are involved in the condition, it can be difficult to draw the TCM diagnosis from the patient's description of Western-style symptoms.

The patient may also be under Western medical treatment, and could be taking medication, chemotherapy or be undergoing procedures such as radiation therapy or surgery. For instance, a woman with breast cancer may be taking tamoxifen, which prevents oestrogen from triggering the growth of the cancer cells. An acupuncturist who does not understand this process may employ points or herbs (such as dong quai) that encourage the body to produce more oestrogen – a serious contraindication.

These days, in most if not all countries, it is rare for a patient to see only an alternative practitioner and eschew conventional medicine entirely. In the West, we cannot practise TCM in a vacuum. In our patients' interest, we must understand enough about conventional medical terms, diagnoses and treatment modalities at least not to harm their health, and at best to optimise it.

In cases where a patient has suffered severe adverse effects at the hands of an alternative medicine practitioner – for instance pneumothorax or transmission of blood-borne disease – courts have rendered judgement on the basis of standards of Western medical practice. The concepts of qi or yin and yang are foreign and irrelevant to the judge or coroner, who decides on the evidence of lab tests, postmortem examinations, etc., what damage has taken place and whether the practitioner is liable. Sometimes an aggrieved patient will blame every subsequent health problem on a treatment even when it is not possible for it to have had that effect. As acupuncturists, the highest standards of ethics require us to have a good knowledge of anatomy, an understanding of medical diagnoses and an ongoing commitment to keep up with advances in medicine.

Although it is obvious that an acupuncturist whose ability is impaired should not be practising at all, even the most competent and conscientious practitioner can make a mistake. Liability insurance protects health professionals in cases of malpractice (errors and omissions). In some jurisdictions it is a legal requirement to purchase malpractice insurance, and most acupuncture colleges or associations offer a group policy. Eventually this may be true everywhere, as registration procedures and legislation governing acupuncture evolve.

Essentially, the practitioner signs over to the insurance agency the right to fight the case, and the agency works on the practitioner's behalf. Although it is embarrassing for any health professional to realise an error or negligence has occurred, it does not help the case to lie about or minimise the facts of the matter. An ethical practitioner assumes full responsibility for the care provided.

Malpractice is not only a question of incompetence. Acupuncturists or TCM practitioners may perform techniques other than acupuncture or moxibustion, for example point injection therapy using herbs or vitamins. Others embed a piece of catgut subcutaneously at certain acupoints. There are also practitioners who open the skin and use vessel forceps to stimulate and suture muscle tissue at an acupoint. Another technique, used to treat people with chronic, severe asthma or allergies, involves cutting the skin and removing a little fatty tissue. In some countries, especially where acupuncturists work in large hospitals, these are normal, common procedures for a TCM practitioner. This is not the case in most Western countries, where often only physicians, nurses and others with special qualifications or permission are allowed to give injections or cause wounds in the body as part of a medical procedure.

Legally, this is a grey area. Acupuncturists are licensed to place needles in people's bodies. What is often unclear is whether this covers using needles to inject herbal preparations, even those processed specifically for this purpose. Practitioners who have been trained in China, Hong Kong, Korea or Japan may not realise, when they relocate to Europe or North America, that this everyday procedure is not allowed. This may be because of licensing regulations or because government health authorities have not approved a certain product for use.

Other prohibitions would involve whether the practitioner has the properly sterile equipment and environment to perform unusual procedures, and whether anaesthesia is required and must therefore be administered by someone who is qualified to do so.

Whether a practitioner has learned one of these more invasive techniques from foreign study or a visiting expert, or may even have acquired many years of experience in its effective use, when moving to a new jurisdiction is wise to check with the licensing body to make sure the practice is permitted. Otherwise the acupuncturist may be open to a charge of malpractice, even if the patient has agreed to the procedure.

Honesty and integrity

Patients have a right to the truth, not only about the risks and benefits of treatments, but also about the practitioner. Ethical practitioners always represent their qualifications honestly, clearly and in a way that is not misleading to patients, the public and to other practitioners. This applies to information given in brochures, advertising, media interviews and educational lectures, as well as to personal communication with patients and their families. Patients have a right to know the fee for a treatment and other services such as sending copies of records to their insurance agency, and, if herbal medicine is indicated, how much extra cost may be incurred.

People come to a practitioner not simply for a diagnosis but also for information as to what to expect, whether the condition is curable, whether the improvement will be dramatic and how long it will take. If expectations are unreasonably raised so that patients look forward to instant relief within days or weeks, later stages of problems experienced on the way toward cure may become highly disappointing. This can damage the reputation of the entire profession, as patients may become discouraged enough to abandon acupuncture altogether and develop negative impressions about TCM.

Another basic principle in the healing professions is the idea of working from a disinterested stance. Disinterest (which is not the same as lack of interest) means that the practitioner refrains from acting on a personal agenda. For instance, in clinics with a herbal pharmacy, practitioners may want to sell the herbal formulas on the shelf and convince themselves that the patient really needs those herbs when in fact the person would be fine without them.

ETHICAL DECISION MAKING IN DAY-TO-DAY PRACTICE

When giving a treatment, the acupuncturist is in a one-to-one relationship with a patient. It is an intimate relationship, in that the practitioner is alone in a room with a person who may be in a vulnerable condition. Ethical practitioners understand it is crucial to create a respectful atmosphere and conduct themselves in a professional manner with individuals.

Since there is a power imbalance in the treatment relationship because the patient is seeking help and relying on the practitioner's expertise, practitioners must promise to respect patients' autonomy. The ideal stance is neutral, which means that practitioners refrain from meeting their own needs through patients. This can be quite subtle, as in a practitioner's need to be heard or validated when really the session is for the *patient* to be heard and validated.

Respecting patients includes allowing them to make their own life decisions. Sometimes practitioners are zealous about their plan to better their patients' health and overstep the patients' autonomy, telling them what would be best to do. It is appropriate to educate and to offer suggestions as opportunities to patients, but not to attempt to control them.

Informed consent

One of the most basic rights of patients is to be adequately informed about the likely benefits and risks of treatment in order to make a decision regarding their own care. As Cantor put it more than 30 years ago, 'The doctrine of informed consent is grounded on the premise that a physician's judgement is subservient to the patient's right of self determination' (Cantor 1973).

Informed consent refers to the practice of educating patients about techniques and possible reactions, and giving them the choice to receive these treatments, refuse them or to stop taking treatment at any time. Patients' freedom of choice is compromised if they are not given enough information to understand fully the risks and benefits of the proposed treatment and decide whether to give or withhold consent. A practitioner has to accept that the patient has full rights to decide against proceeding with the treatment no matter how small a risk of complication. To treat without consent is to commit battery.

Whereas people in many Asian countries have had acupuncture as part of their medical services for generations, and have a full understanding of what to expect, patients who have grown up elsewhere often lack knowledge of acupuncture, compared with their understanding of conventional medicine, so will need more information before they are capable of informed consent.

This could include an information sheet which explains possible side-effects of acupuncture, for example minor bleeding, bruising, pain during treatment, the possibility of fainting as the needles are being inserted, and any adverse reactions after treatment, such as drowsiness or symptoms that get worse before they get better. A brief explanation of common reactions to herbs may also be useful. Also, patients may also need to be told the difference between a desired (even if possibly unpleasant) therapeutic effect and a side-effect. For instance, the practitioner may intend to increase the patient's bowel movements to clear Heat; the patient may think of this as a side-effect.

How much information does a patient need in order for consent to be truly informed? It is impossible to outline every possible complication, especially in complex situations. One definition of sufficient information is that the acupuncturist must provide the patient with enough information for a 'reasonable' person to make a decision regarding therapy. This means that the patient is made aware of the most important and common risks inherent in a properly performed procedure.

This does not mean that the acupuncturist is required to give a patient the details of every treatment. When a patient accepts the therapy, without a detailed explanation of each treatment used, it implies informed consent to receive treatment according to the acupuncturist's best judgement. Nevertheless, practitioners should be aware of the underlying principles as a firm basis for their actions (White et al 2001).

Consent may be given in writing, verbally, or by implication. Patients can imply their consent by preparing themselves for treatment (for instance by climbing on to the treatment bed). If a patient is hesitant in accepting acupuncture treatment and is unable to express concerns, it is a good idea to make sure that explicit verbal consent is obtained. A clear record should be made of the patient's concerns, the practitioner's explanation to alleviate them, and the fact that an explicit verbal consent was asked for and given. If a problem should arise later, a written record that shows the acupuncturist has addressed with this patient any areas of concern or anxiety about the treatment is evidence that the patient has been advised of any potential risks before the treatment began.

In acupuncture there is an array of new procedures and experiences about which a patient should be informed. If using procedures such as moxa cups or electrical stimulation on someone for the first time, it is advisable to tell the patient why this form of treatment has been chosen and what sensations can be expected. The patient's additional consent to any new procedure should be recorded.

The question arises whether the patient's signature should routinely be obtained before acupuncture. In most cases the answer is no, since it cannot be assumed that consent is informed simply because the patient signs a form (White et al 2001). In places where there are licensing bodies, acupuncturists should see whether there are regulations about this. In the absence of such regulations, whether or not to require patients to sign a consent form depends on your judgement of their understanding of acupuncture, their willingness to accept treatment (are they evidently eager to proceed, or do they seem pressured by a spouse or friend?) and your perception of their character. Although I do not believe it is always necessary to have patients sign a form, other practitioners may wish to protect themselves in the event of a later disagreement by obtaining consent in writing.

In the case of a clinic in which interns are practising, I would recommend that patients be provided with a consent form, as the incidence of bruising and other minor adverse reactions may be higher than when procedures are performed by experienced practitioners.

Principles to keep in mind are that the patient should be capable of understanding the information given and forming consent, and that the patient's decision to accept treatment or not be made voluntarily, without coercion by family, friend or health professional.

Regarding children, those 16 years of age and above can be regarded as adults, in terms of their ability to understand information about their treatment and make an informed consent (White et al 2001).

Treatment of children and people with impaired cognitive ability

In Europe and North America, as well as Asia, it is uncommon (though not unheard of) to treat younger children with acupuncture. If it is determined that this is the correct course of action, in addition to the parent's consent I also feel it is imperative that the child receive an explanation of the treatment so that he or she will fully accept it. In my own practice I commonly will do a demonstration needle on the accompanying parent (or teddy bear) first, to help the child be more comfortable.

Patients who have a diminished capacity, such as those who have had severe strokes or are mentally challenged, should be involved in decision making about their treatment to the extent that they are capable. If they do not have the capacity to make decisions about their care, or did not make their wishes known before they became incompetent, consent for care should be sought from a substitute decision maker or caregiver. The caregiver must fully understand and agree to the treatment. In all cases, decisions must be in the best interest of patients and based on what they would want, as far as is known. Lastly, make sure that the patients or their caregivers, or both, clearly understand the financial arrangement of the treatment.

During the consultation and treatment, use simple language so that these patients understand and feel as comfortable as possible. Since it may be difficult for them to verbally communicate sensations and reactions, observe them carefully.

When treating children, or patients with senility or mental disabilities, make sure parents or guardians are present at all times.

Selection and application of treatment

Adequate therapy frequently demands temporary discomfort and risk. In every medical decision, the value of therapy must be weighed against the potential of harm. As therapy is seldom, if ever, risk free, the existence of risk should never in itself be the basis on which to decide whether or not a particular treatment should be given.

However, the acupuncturist's version of the Golden Rule is that the practitioners do not do to their patients what they would not like done to themselves if the roles were reversed. Although they should inform and advise patients what they believe is the best course of action, the patients' opinions must also be respected, even if they conflict with the practitioner's own inclinations. They must appreciate that patients' values may be quite different from their own, whether these are the result of cultural beliefs, varying levels of education or factors that are not immediately obvious. Practitioners should also be sensitive to the patients' social needs with respect to treatments that would be visible to others – for example, ear seeds, cupping marks and the use of points located near the eyes where bruising is likely to arise.

Boundaries and sexual ethics

'Since we work in a physically and sometimes psychologically close manner as healers, it is critical for us to set the guidelines for appropriate behaviour. We occupy positions of power – and sometimes authority – in relation to patients who come to us injured or feeling less than optimal and look to us to help them make changes and get better. And when a person opens to healing, his/her defences are down. It is up to us to provide a safe and secure environment with respect to boundaries so that patients may heal. Regardless of whether we may have been abused ourselves or may feel out of control in our own personal lives, both of which may be entirely possible, it is up to us as professionals to maintain the appropriate boundaries with patients and to seek help for ourselves if we need it' (Brown 1994).

It is a patients' right to refuse to expose parts of the body if they feel uncomfortable doing so. It may be that the person has been left with boundary issues after having experienced childhood abuse or sexual assault. It may simply be that the patient comes from a family or cultural background with strict views about modesty.

Patients who are new to acupuncture will not know how much skin it is appropriate to expose for treatment. A practitioner who asks them to remove more clothing than is necessary may make some patients uncomfortable, especially those of the opposite gender. Europeans tend to be less concerned than North Americans about nudity. If the practitioner is professional and relaxed about nudity, the patient is more likely to feel confidence and trust.

In general, it is proper to request that only the area that will be treated be exposed. Covering with a sheet and perhaps a blanket every part of the patient's body except head, back and limbs is preferable. That means that needling Ren points on the belly or chest, for example, is done with the least amount of skin showing. If a piece of clothing needs to be removed so that a large treatment area is accessible, the patient should be able to undress and dress in private.

Sometimes patients just don't like certain parts of their bodies to be touched, such as their feet. Privacy and a sense of control over how and where one is touched are aspects of feeling safe. Usually if the practitioner tells such patients when he is about to touch them, and asks for permission, the patients will agree.

The flexibility of acupuncture is of great advantage in cases when a patient has issues about a particular body part. As the meridians traverse large portions of the body, it is easy to plan a treatment using distal or other alternative points.

One factor that can make acupuncturists more vulnerable to accusations of inappropriate behaviour is the working environment, which is often unlike the clinical setup of other medical professionals. Sometimes acupuncturists work together as a group, or an acupuncturist shares clinic space with naturopaths, homeopathic practitioners, massage therapists, etc. But more commonly, in Western countries, the acupuncturist and the patient are alone in the clinic, often without even a receptionist outside the door. Clearly, guidelines for appropriate behaviour between acupuncturist and patient are crucial for the protection of both parties in the healing relationship.

Sexual abuse perpetrated by health care professionals is sadly not uncommon. Rules about sexual boundaries are not as clear for acupuncturists as they are for medical doctors, though this is changing as various jurisdictions in the West develop ethical principles for TCM practitioners. See the 'Further reading' list at the end of this section for information on where to find a detailed set of sexual ethics guidelines.

Because acupuncture is such a new field in some parts of the world, non-Asian patients are not always aware of what boundaries and actions performed by the practitioner are appropriate. Some practitioners mix qigong and spiritual work with their acupuncture practice, which may increase the opportunities for improper physical contact and cause patients confusion. For instance, some (though not all) schools of qigong allow the teacher/healer to use his or her hands to push or direct energy along the student/patient's meridians, or even to massage other acupoints along the meridian. An acupuncturist could use such techniques to increase the therapeutic effects. However, problems arise when such therapies involve touching sensitive areas such as sexual parts or a woman's breasts. Even if there is no improper intention on the practitioner's part, this is best avoided.

Cultural differences can also be a factor in sexual ethics. Whereas in some countries tui na may be performed on women's breasts, in the West this constitutes sexual abuse, as some practitioners who have moved to Western countries have discovered to their detriment.

What if a patient requests her practitioner to check out a lump or discomfort in her breast? There are some circumstances in which the acupuncturist may do a physical examination or treatment on a breast: if detailed questioning of the patient has confirmed that the problem has been checked out by a physician and possibly related tests such as a mammogram, that there is clearly a hormonal cause for the cyst or there are signs of infection, or that there is an obvious benefit to placing needles, using moxa or massage on the affected area – for instance in relieving a nursing mother's mastitis. The practitioner never works on a patient's nipple.

As for touching other areas such as the vulva, anus or perineum, there is no need for an acupuncturist to perform an internal examination. There are, of course, many acupoints on and around sexual parts. However, there are many substitute points that can be employed for these, as well as points on the same meridian but farther away that can be used effectively. Very rarely, there is no choice in the matter – for instance points used in treatment of haemorrhoids. For the protection of patient and practitioner, it is a good idea to treat sensitive areas only when a third party is present, preferably a relative or friend of the patient, but if necessary the receptionist or another practitioner.

When treating parts of the body close to sensitive areas, such as the chest, lower abdomen or buttocks, and the patients' clothing or draping needs to be moved, their permission must be requested, and their preferences must be respected. Sometimes newer practitioners will try to lighten the atmosphere and cover their own embarrassment in such situations by joking, for instance, about their ineptitude in undoing the hooks on a brassiere. This is inappropriate and unprofessional, as are remarks about the patient's body. There is no place for flirting or otherwise creating a sexually suggestive atmosphere in a treatment context.

The practitioner uses only the hands to palpate and only the hands and elbows to perform massage or acupressure. In addition, the knee, lateral aspect of the hip and lower leg are the only parts of the practitioner's body to be used for bracing; the front of the pelvis is not acceptable.

Another major area of ethical concern arises in forming romantic/sexual relationships with patients. Since a practitioner is in a position of trust, it is unethical to begin a non-therapeutic relationship with a patient. Existing codes of ethics clearly state that practitioners do not exploit their patients' vulnerabilities for their own interests, whether these are sexual, emotional, social, political, financial or in any other way. If a personal relationship develops, the practitioner must stop treating this patient and refer the person to an associate. The relationship must be fully consensual on both sides; there must never be coercion by the practitioner. If both parties are interested in pursuing an emotional/sexual relationship, it should commence some time after treatments have ended. Some codes of ethical conduct suggest 3 months as the acceptable minimum length of time between the end of a treatment relationship and the beginning of a romantic one.

Even friendships can be tricky between practitioners and patients. When treating someone with whom they have a social acquaintanceship, practitioners must be careful to keep the treatment within a professional context and atmosphere, and maintain a clear separation from the social setting. In other words, if you go to someone's house for dinner, and are asked to do acupuncture on the host, it is probably best to suggest the person make an appointment for treatment at your clinic or at least a separate house call.

Confidentiality

The information given to a medical practitioner by a patient is given in confidence and is not for publication or disclosure without the patient's consent. Confidentiality is an important issue in the health field. Many people come to a TCM practitioner by word of mouth; therefore, it is especially important not to disclose information about anyone, even to their friends.

Unless a child is involved, or two people ask to be treated at the same time, the acupuncturist should not share information even with family members without the patient's permission. An exception may be when a family member has a serious illness, such as cancer, when all members would like to be informed and involved in helping that person.

Practitioners and receptionists may need to be reminded that any conversations with patients, either in person or on the phone, regarding the reasons for their treatment should be conducted quietly so as not to be overheard by others. And it is also important to remember that, when communicating with professional colleagues about a case, care should be taken not to refer to patients' names or any identifying details within the hearing of others, such as in the coffee shop or the elevator.

Patient records should be kept in such a way that they are not accessible to the public, or left on a counter even for a few minutes where others can see them. These days, records are frequently stored on computers, and security is an increasingly serious issue. Access to these should be available only to authorised people, using codes or passwords. It is advisable to make back-up copies and to store them in a safe, secure place, preferably somewhere else.

Situations often arise in which patients request practitioners to send their private data to insurance companies, lawyers or governmental agencies. If insurance claims are involved, it is important to be sure an information release is signed by the patient before sending records to the third party. The signed information release should be kept in the patient's file, with a note of the date the request was received and the date the information was sent out. The practitioner should keep all the original records, and send out copies only. A copy may be given to the patient as well. If these records are ever read out in court, it may be useful to have added short explanatory notes that indicate the names of points, herbs, techniques of stimulation and anything else that may be unclear to someone with no knowledge of Chinese medicine.

A practitioner who writes an article that includes a case history should make sure identifying details such as name and address are concealed.

Special issues of confidentiality and ethics

David Ip RAc, DTCM, DAc

TCM practitioners may be asked to treat conditions associated with socially controversial lifestyles, including multiple sexual partners, certain trades or professions, substance abuse, addictive behaviour, etc. Several aspects of controversial lifestyles are relevant to health practitioners.

First, confidentiality rules protect patients' disclosures. However, more than normal efforts might sometimes be needed to protect privacy. Leakage of personal lifestyle information, such as sexual orientation, could jeopardise a person's employment or employability, or their family or social relationships. Lifestyles associated with shorter lifespans could affect their insurability. Information about employment in some industries such as biochemicals, manufacturing or entertainment could bring damaging attention from media, activists or other areas, and most importantly could affect the patient's willingness to get treatment. It is essential to demonstrate explicitly that the client's confidentiality is assured. This could be done by referring to your professional organisation's code of ethics verbally or on the consent form.

In some cases, there may be lifestyle circumstances in which the practitioner faces a confidentiality dilemma. An example is a patient with a transmissible or contagious disease whose lifestyle or activities may jeopardise others (e.g. through body fluid exposure, food industry occupation, health services, etc.). If a patient with a transmissible disease discloses potential exposure to others, you may be ethically (and in some jurisdictions legally) obliged to disclose the danger either to those at risk, such as family members, or to suitable authorities. A patient whose condition is not transmissible to others can also present a public danger that outweighs the right to privacy; one example would be someone who could have an epileptic seizure while operating a vehicle.

Discussing such a situation with a patient can be awkward or frightening depending on the patient's volatility. Often, the best course is to encourage patients to take responsibility by disclosing their condition to people who might be at risk, and to refrain from hazardous activity.

Discussing difficult subjects

In communicating with and treating patients, subjects may arise that are difficult to discuss owing to social, legal, medical or emotional circumstances. In these cases, there is no single simple approach. Thinking about potential situations before they arise can help the practitioner avoid some of the awkwardness or a possibly inappropriate response.

Substance abuse, overindulgence in sex, exposure to multiple sexual partners, hazardous work, etc., are all topics that may be difficult to broach, especially when an open rapport has not yet developed between patient and practitioner. There is an important distinction between passing judgement on how someone contracted an illness and advocating a healthy lifestyle or a change in such activities. In addressing the person's lifestyle, the practitioner must maintain objectivity and non-judgement so that the patient feels secure enough to disclose information necessary for an accurate assessment. If patients are willing to make a life change, you can help turn their discomfort with their lifestyle into a positive force. For example, addiction can be effectively treated with TCM. People successfully treated can eventually become powerful advocates both for TCM and for social improvement once their lives are balanced and moderate, whereas being met with exposure or condemnation in their initial encounters with an acupuncturist could be emotionally devastating or destroy their motivation to seek help.

Personal biases may affect the willingness of health care professionals to treat certain people. Practitioners must be aware of their own biases or experiences that may limit treatment effectiveness. For example, family illness related to pesticides may prevent you from empathising with a patient who works in the pesticide industry. If you are uncomfortable with a patient's lifestyle to the extent that treating them compromises your own personal values, or your own background compromises your ability to provide effective treatment, you are still bound ethically to protect the patient's privacy and to inform them that you cannot adequately care for them.

ABUSE

In the course of assessment or treatment, a patient may disclose to a practitioner that abuse has occurred. Disclosures in certain situations are addressed by the law; be familiar with the legislation regarding your obligations. If the abuse involves minors or dependents (e.g. a shut-in resident), it must be reported to legal authorities. If the persons involved are not minors but the event is recent and unaddressed or ongoing, it may be necessary to report it especially if someone is in danger. If you suspect that the patient is about to disclose something requiring legal action, you should advise them that by law you cannot guarantee confidentiality. However, you can do everything possible to find an appropriate legal and supportive course of action.

In assessment interviews, there may be disclosure of events that the patient has previously addressed or do not require third party intervention. You may need to determine whether the impact of the abuse is a factor in the person's current health (e.g. depression, fear, anger, insecurity, etc.). In this case, you must respond to the person's trust with care, respect and compassion. Patients might be willing to discuss the events if they think it is necessary for the treatment, but if details are unnecessary then discussion may lead to a painful or unnecessarily awkward atmosphere. It may be helpful to explain how their emotional or mental traumas can affect their physiological health (endogenous pathogenic factors); this can give validity to their experience without having to revisit it, and brings the focus to their current health, which is your professional domain. (Some codes of ethics clearly state that even when the practitioner suspects a history of abuse, but the patient hasn't disclosed it, it is not up to the practitioner to confront the patient with this interpretation.)

Again, if your own background might hinder your treatment or equanimity, you might need to inform patients that you cannot effectively help them. Sometimes, simply offering a tissue is all that is necessary to show suitable compassion and care. At other times, if the events are still unresolved, it may be necessary to help patients find a professional counsellor or other qualified therapist. If patients explicitly request help during a disclosure, you must be clear about the professional qualifications you hold (or do not hold) to address their concern.

Another aspect of disclosures is that others involved may still be in the patient's life, or may even be known to you. Unless your patient wishes to address the experience with you explicitly, or unless there is a potential threat to someone, your job is to treat your patient with utmost confidentiality, which extends to the other persons involved.

In any questionable situation, it is advisable to seek legal counsel regarding your obligations.

SUICIDE IDEATION

Depression at its extreme may encompass the desire for an end to something, usually some kind of suffering. Although TCM practitioners treat many aspects of depression, if someone is thinking about suicide (ideation) you may be required to act quickly, possibly without time to reflect. If patients threaten suicide, talk about wanting to die or deliberately injure themselves, do not ignore it. If you believe patients are a danger to themselves or to someone else, you may have to inform someone. Tell them that you are obliged to get help for them and encourage them to do so themselves. Unless you are trained as a suicide intervention counsellor, you must not take it upon yourself to counsel such patients. However, there are several steps you can take to address immediate concerns.

Guidelines for responding to suicide ideation

—Stay calm and listen.
—Let them talk about their feelings.
—Be accepting; do not judge.
—Ask if they have suicidal thoughts.
—Take threats seriously.
—Don't swear secrecy; tell someone. Persons to contact could be family, friends, clergy, teachers, counsellors, doctors, crisis lines, mental health services or hospital emergency departments.

END-OF-LIFE ISSUES

Many TCM patients suffer terminal diseases or the increasingly unbearable conditions of deteriorating health. In Western countries, medical doctors and specialists usually provide treatment at the end of life (palliative care). But as TCM becomes more regulated and integrated into the health sector, practitioners will find themselves encountering more end-of-life situations. The era of life-saving and life-preserving technologies has given many people the hope that once-terminal conditions might be survived indefinitely. Furthermore, the advent of the information age has opened a door to patients' unprecedented understanding of their own conditions, and the impetus to take control of their own health care. Thus many are refusing to accept terminal diagnoses and are turning to alternative practices, such as TCM, in the hope of a different prognosis. Conventional health care providers, family members and others around the patient may feel that practices like TCM provide false hope or unreasonably drain a desperate person's finances.

It is essential that the TCM practitioner give a professionally supportable prognosis for the desired outcome. A compassionate, unhurried discussion with the patient and family members is crucial, in order to be clear about everyone's hopes and expectations. The patient may be under pressure from many people. You must provide information in an understandable way without antagonising those closest to the patient. Your obligation is to do what is best for the patient. Stress, medication and the unfamiliar terminology of TCM can make this discussion difficult for a patient with a terminal illness to grasp. The following guidelines may help:

Guidelines for handling end-of-life issues

—Take a lot of time to be sure patients and their supporters understand you.
—Write information down for people to be able to read over and over again.
—If language is a concern, ask for a translator.
—Give patients time and privacy to discuss the information with others (a few minutes or a few days), and to come back with questions.
—Offer to meet with their physician to discuss options so that they do not feel torn between different practitioners and practices.

Some patients may come who have accepted their prognosis but seek relief from pain, dysfunction or the side-effects of conventional medical treatments. These conditions increasingly detract from quality of life and may lead to thinking about suicide, do-not-resuscitate orders, advance directives, surrogate decision makers, etc. Significant stresses surround these literally life-and-death decisions, robbing these patients of energy and time at the end of their life. TCM has a particular role to offer those struggling with end-of-life decisions. The Gall Bladder governs decision making; fear and fright affect the Kidneys, and anger upsets the Liver. Treatment of endogenous pathogenic factors according to TCM principles may help to calm patients and clear their minds at a time of great emotional upheaval and huge decisions.

A TCM practitioner may be called upon to discuss not only a person's health condition, but also their values, desires, fears and spiritual beliefs. It requires compassion, tact, humility, empathy and professional competence. It may require interaction with those caregiving and keeping vigil for the patient in their transition. A very good guide is to think how we would want our loved ones to be treated at the same time in their lives.

Ownership and usage of treatment records   *Hong Zhen Zhu*

Who owns the treatment records – the acupuncturist or the patient? This is not an easy question to answer. When a patient is moving to a new city, it is certainly appropriate to send copies of the file to the new practitioner, if requested.

But what if the patient just wants to see them? The tricky issue is that practitioners' case notes serve several functions, not the least of which is helping their self-defence if a dispute later arises about, for example, whether they recommended that patients see their medical doctor. However patient's right to access and copies of medical records has been upheld in several court decisions (Heifetz 1994).

The self-protective intentions of practitioners or the fear of disclosing errors does not in any way outweigh patients' right to the actual treatment record, or at least to copies of these records. It also includes the right to know to whom that data has been revealed or who has access to it. Patients' desire to see their records is valid regardless of their reasons for wanting to do so.

Plans should be made for the disposition of patients' files in the event of the early or unexpected death of the practitioner.

CONSULTATION, REFERRAL AND PROFESSIONAL RELATIONSHIPS

Another important issue in acupuncture ethics involves realising when it is appropriate to advise a patient to stop coming to you and to see a family doctor or medical specialist instead. All practitioners have a responsibility to know the limits of what they can do, and advise patients accordingly.

To illustrate this, a man once came to me for treatment of jaundice, saying he had heard acupuncture and herbs could treat this successfully. If he had also reported feeling pain, I would have suspected gallstones or some infection and treated him accordingly. However, I knew that painless jaundice is a serious warning symptom of possible bile duct cancer, and urged him to see his physician immediately. Treating him with acupuncture at that time would have been a major breach of professional ethics.

Patients' health needs and rights are best served when we respect and value the contributions of other health care providers and work in cooperation with them.

Ethical acupuncturists are aware of their own limitations in skill or knowledge, and are prepared to put patients' best interests ahead of their ego. If, despite the practitioner's best efforts, a patient's condition is still not improving, the time may come when it is appropriate to refer the person to a different or more senior practitioner. Patients should be able to have faith that their practitioners will not attempt anything beyond their ability and will seek consultation if necessary.

The new practitioner to whom a patient is being referred should be supplied with adequate information about the person's TCM diagnosis, treatments, results and the length of time the original acupuncturist has been seeing the person. It is also important to be clear about what type of help is being requested from the consulting practitioner and whether this is temporary or long term.

If you have a patient referred to you, it is wise to inquire about the history of the person's condition and any previous experiences with acupuncture. After the consultation and treatment, make sure that you understand whether or not you are expected to see this patient again, or if the person is returning to the original practitioner. Ask both the patient and the previous practitioner.

When you plan to move to another city or to take a holiday for longer than 4 weeks, it is your responsibility to plan for the care of your patients. This may involve letters of referral or making other arrangements for them.

Refusing or withdrawing treatment

The idea of 'firing' a patient is a sensitive issue that is still undergoing discussion in the profession. In general medical practice, the practitioner has the right not to accept someone as a patient, and also has the right to resign from the management of a case, but is not allowed to 'abandon' the patient. This means that it is the practitioners' responsibility to make arrangements for another qualified person to assume the care of patients, before withdrawing their services. The acupuncturist may also have an associate monitor and care for a patient during vacation or while away for educational purposes as long as the latter has been informed.

In order to avoid getting into legal trouble for abandonment, the practitioner is expected to have good reasons for denying or withdrawing services. These may include having no room in the practice for new patients, evidence of unreasonable demands by a patient, a patient who is uncooperative and refuses to follow prescribed treatment, or in some cases non-payment of fees agreed to by the patient. The practitioner should inform the patient of the reasons for withdrawal of treatment, give sufficient notice to find another qualified practitioner and may refer the patient to an appropriate practitioner.

Differences of opinion with other TCM practitioners

David Ip RAc, DTCM, DAc

There are dozens of schools of thought on the practice and ethics of TCM. The body of knowledge is rich, diverse and continually increasing; certainly no one person could grasp all aspects of it.

Each of us is also unique, with the sum of our experiences, training, perceptions and values affecting our understanding and practice of TCM. These differences are strengths in our profession. However, ways of expressing the differences can be a weakness. In ancient China, practitioners were typically independent, sharing knowledge when they might meet, but each responsible for his own conduct rather than relying on a single regulatory body. In North America and Europe, standardisation and regulation have been foundations of professional medicine for centuries. In Europe, North America, Australia and New Zealand, TCM is developing into a respected coordinated profession, but occasions arise when one practitioner believes that another's opinion or action is erroneous, is not in the patient's best interests, harms the profession, or even is not relevant to TCM.

The traditional Chinese concept of 'face' would prevent people from making public accusations and broadcasting internal disharmony. Chinese culture is rich with the art of subtly demonstrating disagreements or differences without involving the whole community. However, the power of politics in our modern-day institutions, departments and committees has drawn people into publicly praising or condemning opinions in frustration, to gain public support, or to intimidate those 'opposed'. These differences of opinion spill over into the public arena as unprofessionalism, incompetence and confusion.

Actions considered to be unprofessional include criticising other practitioners or practices in public (including to patients), attempting to benefit oneself at the public expense of another and conduct beneath the dignity of the profession or its professional bodies.

Unprofessional conduct may be easy or difficult to comment upon depending on whether patients are involved. For example, most practitioners are members of some professional organisation with rules of conduct. Members who volunteer their time in the organisation leadership are generally expected to refrain from using their positions in advertising, etc. Practitioners can be told directly that they are clearly violating rules or regulations, and patient care is unlikely to be affected. The approach might be quite different if patients are involved. For example, selling services or products that claim outrageous benefits has been considered unethical and unprofessional for millennia in both TCM and conventional Western medicine. There are numerous irresponsible claims of TCM treatments for sexual prowess that ignore the fundamental TCM principle of treating the person, and many practitioners regard making such claims as unprofessional. However, to denounce publicly a distributor of such products may undermine patient trust in TCM and prompt those with genuine sexual dysfunction to forgo professional and effective treatment including an explanation of the dangers of overindulgence.

Incompetence on the part of a TCM practitioner includes inappropriate treatment, unreasonable claims of efficacy, prolonged treatment of unresponsive conditions, failure to answer reasonable patient questions, treatment outside the scope of training, etc. Incompetence is very difficult to address, especially as professional training is required to evaluate a practitioner, and there are many grey areas. Most professional organisations review questions of incompetence behind closed doors, so that sensitive issues can be addressed fairly and thoroughly before issuing a conclusion publicly. Although intended to protect the privacy of practitioners before passing judgement, often closed-door reviews are denounced as an attempt at secrecy. Some practitioners decline to cooperate with such reviews because of concerns over conflicts, partisanship and other differences of opinion.

Part of the evolution of self-regulating TCM bodies in the West is the requirement for effective, fair methods to address questions of competence. In the meantime, the approach in some jurisdictions will remain that of the doctor in traditional China – one of individual conscience. When a practitioner strongly and sincerely believes that another practitioner's conduct is wrong or potentially harmful, the issue should first be raised privately with that practitioner in a professional and courteous manner. Personal likes and dislikes have no place in a discussion of professional conduct or competence. If the practitioner is not responsive, you may be ethically obliged to bring the concern to the practitioner's registering body.

Confusion is common throughout the health care world as personal and professional opinions bombard patients from all sides. There are numerous different therapies and therapists in most large urban centres now, and the public may have little awareness of the difference between a certified profession and a non-standardised practice. For many people, TCM is seen as the same as any 'new' theory, rather than a discipline with thousands of years of accumulated and tested methodology. Those who practise a therapeutic form of counselling or treatment have a professional obligation to advise each client which aspects are TCM and which are not. If the clients are interested in TCM treatment alone, they might reject the entire practice on the basis of disliking the therapy being offered. Practitioners have an ethical responsibility to present their practice based on sound principles, repeatable results and openness to scrutiny.

Finally, expressing an opinion can be very intimidating. Differences of opinion may be directed toward a single practitioner, or to a group with something in common. In some jurisdictions, the TCM community can number fewer than a dozen in many towns and cities, to perhaps 200 in larger urban centres. This is usually a fraction of the number of physicians working in most large cities. Significant differences can easily involve most or all TCM practitioners in a given community. Some opinions, especially when expressed in public, may be subject to libel and slander laws. Expressing differences of opinions in public has divided health care organisations, given rise to political factions and, at its extreme, has been known to end in violence.

The right to express an opinion carries also the responsibility for the consequences of that opinion. If you are going to express a contrary opinion in public, ask yourself whether it will help a patient or the profession. If the interests of the patient are put first, and if the good of the profession is at stake, it may be necessary to act. To protect professionalism requires patience, compassion and courage.

References

Branch WT Jr 2000 The ethics of caring and medical education. Academic Medicine 75:127

Brown SD 1994 Sexual ethics guidelines. Acupuncture Association of BC Winter Newsletter Feb: p 7–11

Cantor N 1973 A patient's decision to decline life-saving medical treatment. Rutgers Law Review 26:12

Heifetz MD 1994 The patient–doctor relationship. Health education: knowledge from the West. Universal Science Publishing House, Beijing, p 138-159

Kaptchuk TJ 2002 Acupuncture: theory, efficacy, and practice. Annals of Internal Medicine 136:374-383

Lo B 1998 Ethical issues in clinical medicine. In: Harrison's principles of internal medicine. 14th edn. McGraw-Hill, New York. p 6-8

MacPherson H, Thomas K, Walters S et al 2001 A prospective survey of adverse events and treatment reactions following 34 000 consultations with professional acupuncturists. Acupuncture in Medicine 19(2):93-102

NIH Consensus Conference 1998 Acupuncture. Journal of the American Medical Association 280(17):1518-1524

White A, Cummings M, Hopwood V et al 2001 Informed consent for acupuncture – an information leaflet developed by consensus. Acupuncture in Medicine 19(2):123-129

Further reading

Many countries, licensing/certification bodies and educational institutions have codes of ethics for acupuncturists and other Chinese medicine practitioners. They generally cover most of the same issues. The following are examples of organisations with well-developed codes, for those who wish to refer to them.

In the United Kingdom:
British Acupuncture Council
Codes of professional conduct and safe practice
Contact: 63 Jeddo Road, London W129HQ
tel: 020 8735 0400; fax: 020 8735 0404; email: ethics@acupuncture.org.uk, info@acupuncture.org.uk; website: www.acupuncture.org.uk
British Medical Acupuncture Society (BMAS)
12 Marbury House, Higher Whitley, Warrington, Cheshire WA4 4QW
tel: + 44 (0) 1925 730727; email: admin@medical-acupuncture.org.uk; website: www.medical-acupuncture.co.uk
The Acupuncture Society
163 Northwood Way, Northwood, Middlesex HA6 1RA
general enquiries: + 44 (0) 1923 822 972; email: info@acupuncturesociety.org.uk; website: www.acupuncturesociety.org.uk

In Canada:
At the time of writing, there is no national code of ethics, and only a few provinces have registration bodies. British Columbia has the most developed system, which is becoming the model in other Canadian provinces, so its code of ethics is given here as a reference.

College of Traditional Chinese Medicine Practitioners and Acupuncturists of British Columbia (CTCMA)
Code of ethics for registrants /standards of practice for registrants
Contact: 2nd Floor, 5050 Kingsway, Burnaby, BC, Canada V5H 4H2
tel: 604-638-3108; fax: 604-683-3103; email: info@ctcma.bc.ca; website: www.ctcma.bc.ca

In the United States:
National Certification Commission for Acupuncture and Oriental Medicine (NCCAOM)
Code of ethics (revised May 2004)
Contact: 11 Canal Center Plaza, Suite 300, Alexandria, Virginia 22314
tel: 703-548-9004; fax: 703-548-9079; email: info@nccaom.org; website:
    www.nccaom.org

In Australia:
Australian Acupuncture and Chinese Medicine Association Ltd. (AACMA)
Code of ethics
Contact: (mailing address) PO Box 5142 West End Queensland, 4101
Registered national office: Suite 5, 28 Gladstone Rd., Highgate Hill, Brisbane,
    Queensland 4101, Australia
tel: +61 (0)7 3846 5866; fax: +61 (0)7 3846 5276; email: aacma@acupuncture.org.au;
    website: www.acupuncture.org.au

Interpersonal skills with patients

7

Truly gifted healers have skills that go beyond the mastery of TCM technique. They are also part psychologist, part teacher, and part coach. The acupuncturist's role is not to judge or harangue a patient about bad health habits, but to offer information and encouragement based on an understanding of each patient's needs. Practitioners who have well-developed interpersonal skills make their patients feel comfortable, understood and cared for. As we know, such intangible elements can have a profound influence on the healing process.

TCM fits well with a growing desire on the part of many people to participate in their health care. Patients are more likely to comply with their practitioner's treatment suggestions when they understand what is being done to their bodies and why. It is a balancing act between giving patients enough information so they understand how TCM can help them, but not so much that they are confused and overwhelmed. Practitioners have to be confident enough that patients feel assured they're in competent hands, but take care not to convey the idea that they can perform miracles.

Don't rush. While you don't want to give the impression you know everything, learn how to look as though you know what the patient is talking about even when you don't. Then go and look it up right away. It is important to have good, well-organised reference materials, as well as a list of other professionals – not just TCM practitioners – you can call for more information. (Of course this means you have to be prepared to help others when they call you.)

An equally important part of communication is the practitioner's ability to *listen* to the patient's feedback. For example, a point is effective only once the sensation of 'de qi' has been felt by both patient and practitioner. The sensation of de qi may be uncomfortable for some patients; preparing them for this strange feeling beforehand will help them to accept it. After a few treatments, most patients will guide practitioners as to their preferred strength of stimulation. Some patients are initially so afraid of needles that it is necessary to use tui na, acupressure, ear beads or herbal medicine before gradually introducing them to needling.

People who are looking for a 'quick fix' will be disappointed if their symptoms are not relieved with one treatment. Remember to explain that the effects of acupuncture are cumulative. Help patients to understand that improvements may not be great initially, but that over time and after several treatments they will notice the benefits.

Write down lifestyle change suggestions for patients, as they are often drowsy after a treatment and will forget what you have said. Have a notepad with your name on it or use a letterhead. Patients can stick it on their fridge as a reminder. And they will remember you the next time they need help.

Chinese medicine is based on the Taoist concept of humans existing between Heaven and Earth. In practical terms, this means an inclusive approach with patients and their families involved in dietary changes, exercising, meditating, learning how to make herbal decoctions and providing emotional support. As a practitioner, this means that your role is as an educator as well as a member of the healing circle for each patient. A family consultation may be necessary when initiating a treatment plan, or later, when you see that it would be beneficial. An acupuncturist does not assume a central role, because all team members are considered to be equal participants. If anyone is central, it is the patient.

Especially in countries where acupuncture is relatively new, it is imperative to share information about it, to educate people, and to allow and welcome everyone's questions concerning it. It is not appropriate for practitioners to take offence when people inquire about their training, expertise and equipment. Patients need – and have the right – to feel safe. Open acceptance of all their questions helps to build trust and mutual respect in the therapeutic relationship.

TEACHING PATIENTS ABOUT ACUPUNCTURE AND TCM

This section presents the most common questions patients ask their acupuncturist. It is helpful to consider and develop answers in advance, when not pressured by time or concentrating on giving a treatment.

Patients will typically come in with a list of things to ask about. The practitioner who is listening carefully should be able to select the most pressing concerns. The way you then answer is important so that patients know you have heard them, understood them and satisfactorily addressed their major issues.

The greatest numbers of questions usually come up during the first treatment or two. If a telephone conversation with a prospective patient suggests that a lot of information is needed because acupuncture is totally new to the person, you can invite the patient to come in and talk for 15 minutes at the end of your day in order to answer questions and to provide an opportunity to decide whether or not this form of treatment is of interest. Many practitioners offer this kind of short consultation at no charge. Incidentally, 80% of the time these people do make an appointment at the end of their talk with you. Always, as we say in Chinese, 'give them a ladder to get out', that is, a gracious way to go or simply not to decide at that moment. You can tell them that they are free to phone with more questions, or to discuss things with their families before they get back to you.

As you know, practitioners are dealing with human beings who have multiple factors in their lives. If people do not make an appointment the same day, it does not mean that they are not interested. They may have to arrange for babysitters, work schedules, check their extended medical plan coverage, or finish their school assignments.

From a business perspective, of course, it is better that they do make an appointment. If you have many callers who do not, a self-evaluation of your telephone skills may be in order; do you sound knowledgeable, professional, interested and energetic? There is more information about this in Section Three.

Explaining acupuncture and TCM

It is usually a challenge to explain the basic concepts and system of TCM and acupuncture to people who are not from Asian backgrounds. There are many areas of confusion for patients, especially in understanding how we use terminology, such as the names of organs, differently from the Western medical concepts. Sometimes giving patients a little bit of information – such as saying the Liver is 'tight' – gives rise to misunderstandings that, if not cleared up, can cause patients worry and distress, and damage the credibility of individual acupuncturists and our profession.

Whereas some patients are eager to learn more about this holistic form of medicine, most just want and need a short explanation of their condition in terms the average person can understand. Define any new terms you may introduce, such as yin, yang, qi and meridian; even though these are natural to your vocabulary they may well be foreign to patients. However, you can waste a lot of time trying to explain concepts that took you years to understand. In many cases it is acceptable to say something like 'I am balancing your energy, which will relieve your symptoms' rather than go into a long technical explanation. 'Liver yang rising' can be described as energy flowing upwards into the head, causing symptoms such as headache, dizziness or insomnia.

Having spent years struggling with this myself, I eventually wrote a book to try to bridge the gap between Chinese medicine and the Western mind. Many students and practitioners have told me that it is extremely helpful in giving them simple ways to explain TCM and acupuncture (Zhu 2003).

Practitioners have to choose vocabulary carefully, especially when treating people of other cultural backgrounds who may have a different understanding of certain words. One example is a word like 'hypochondrium'. It is a legitimate anatomical term for the area just below the anterior ribcage. However, I once learned the hard way that it is not a good word to use in explaining the situation to a patient! Many people will assume you are implying that their symptoms are all in their heads.

Each practitioner will, over time, develop personal ways of answering questions, but the following suggestions are a place to start.

Common questions about acupuncture and TCM

How does acupuncture work?

Ask patients whether they are familiar with TCM, which will give you a clue as to the level of information required. Someone new to acupuncture may be satisfied with this short description: the human body contains a system of pathways, or meridians, through which vital energy, called qi, travels. When the free flow of qi is blocked or out of balance, illness is the result. When needles are placed in one or more of several hundred points on the skin that connect to the meridians, it stimulates the flow of energy, which seems to trigger various self-healing mechanisms in the body. The application of heat or acupressure to these points also stimulates energy flow, but needling is the most effective.

In terms of Western medicine, acupuncture can change levels of hormones, release endorphins and affect counts of red and white blood cells. Although modern scientific studies are only beginning to give us an idea of the physiological mechanisms involved, one piece of evidence that acupuncture works is that it is used successfully on babies and animals, who cannot be influenced by the placebo effect.

Does acupuncture hurt?

When done by a properly trained practitioner, it should not be painful. But we do want the patient to feel what we call de qi, or a good needle sensation, which is a sign that the treatment will have an effect. The patient can be reassured that the sensation is usually more achy in quality rather than sharply painful. It also helps to explain that some points are more sensitive than others, and that the sensations may be stronger at various times, depending on the person's condition and what kind of treatment is being done. You can also mention that you can modify the treatment if necessary, and that you know techniques to make needle insertion more comfortable, so you do want to hear feedback from the patient and do not expect him or her to endure pain.

Do you use disposable needles?

This seems to be a really basic question. However, patients are often concerned about stories they have read in the newspaper regarding untrained or unregulated 'practitioners' who are causing disease or infection with contaminated needles. They may need to be assured that you practise sterile procedures at all times. This information can also be included in a brochure.

What does it mean when you look at my tongue and feel my pulse?

The tongue and the pulse are special and important diagnostic tools in Chinese medicine. The appearance of the tongue and the different kinds and qualities of pulse indicate any imbalances in the flow of energy through the various organ systems. In classical Chinese medical philosophy, yin and yang are the two fundamental and opposing energies in the universe and therefore in the body. Each organ system has its own ideal proportion of yin and yang energies; too much or too little of either results in an excess or deficiency of Heat, Cold, Dampness, Dryness, etc., which causes symptoms. When we diagnose the energy imbalances, we can design treatments that reduce, increase or unblock energy where needed.

How old is this system of Chinese medicine?

It is four to five thousand years old and the principles and goals have remained constant through time. Acupuncture was used by numerous 19th century American physicians and it is now recognised by established medical organisations in practically every part of the world, including the National Institutes of Health (US) and the World Health Organization.

How did people discover acupuncture and herbs?

It was probably by chance that people first discovered eating certain plants or having bamboo thorns or sharp stones pressed at certain points on their body helped to ease pains resulting from a difficult life of finding food, making shelters and having children. Generation after generation then refined and added to this knowledge of herbs and points eventually to develop the complex system of today.

What is chinese herbology and how does it differ from Western?

What TCM calls 'herbs' may be made from plants, animal parts or minerals. Unlike in Western herbal practice, where a certain herb is used to treat a particular set of symptoms, Chinese herbs are prescribed according to the way their special characteristics balance energy in various organs or meridians. Prescriptions tend to have many different herbs in them because each has its own job; some modify the effects of the others that would be too strong on their own. When it comes to raw herbal preparations, each prescription is tailored to the individual's needs and condition – taking into account the patient's age, gender, physical condition and immediate symptoms. If herbal decoctions are too inconvenient to prepare, or unpalatable, there are usually choices of patent medicines that will work.

In recent years, many patients have become concerned about Chinese medicine's use of herbal preparations made from the parts of endangered animals. A properly trained practitioner does not use these. There are equally effective alternatives.

Common questions about your training and background

What made you decide to be an acupuncturist?

Many practitioners have a personal story to share about a health problem of their own or of someone close to them that was relieved by acupuncture. Patients appreciate and respond to your passion for your work.

What was your training in acupuncture?

Describe your schooling experience, the background of your instructors, how old your college is, and any apprenticeships or studying abroad you have done.

Common questions about the patient's own condition

Do you treat people with my condition with acupuncture?

You may not have treated this condition before but you *know* you are competent to treat it. If you're not sure exactly how to proceed, it is fair for you to give the patient a general balancing treatment and then research more specific details for the next visit.

What does my TCM diagnosis mean?

If, for example, the diagnosis is a Kidney yin deficiency, reassure the patient that you do not necessarily mean that the Kidney itself has a problem, but that the overall pattern of energy in the body is out of balance, in this example the moistening and nourishing energy in particular. This bears repeating: patients will need to hear that Chinese medicine's use of organ names is nearly always different from the Western meaning. This will also help prevent misunderstandings with the patient's medical practitioner. Patients have been known to rush off to their physician and demand tests to check the allegedly dysfunctional organ.

How many treatments do I need, and how often?

Of course this is individual, but in general depends on whether a patient's condition is in the acute, chronic, or maintenance category. Please refer to the section on treatment planning in Section Three for more specific guidelines. You can say that, during the acute phase, treatments are more frequent to ease the initial problem and help the patient feel better faster. Reassure your patient that each treatment builds on the effects of the previous one. As symptoms improve, treatments will not be as frequent, but will still be needed at certain intervals to maintain the changes and to address any underlying problems or imbalances. Even when people are feeling better, an occasional 'tune-up' with acupuncture will keep their immune system strong and their energy balanced, to avoid illness.

May my friend or family member accompany me during treatment?

Most of the time we treat patients alone, even at the first consultation. However, there are circumstances in which it is appropriate for a friend or family member to accompany a patient. For example, it would be fine for an elderly person to be accompanied by an adult child who takes care of the parent, and who has researched their parent's condition and wants to understand how to help according to Chinese medicine. Others with physical disabilities or extreme weakness may need someone to assist them even with getting on and off the treatment table; normally these assistants remain throughout the treatment. If they ask too many questions, you may tell them that the patient needs quiet to benefit fully from the treatment. Unless there is a pressing need to have them in the room, spouses or friends should be asked to sit in the waiting area before the consultation begins.

After the treatment, it is a good idea to invite the caregiver in from the waiting area in order to explain your treatment plan, your analysis of the situation and how they can assist the healing process at home by preparing food, encouraging exercise, massaging or cooking herbs. Do not forget to ask them if they have any questions to ask you! This is a good opportunity to expand your practice. Normally this is also an appropriate time to give them your pamphlet.

During my treatment, should I discontinue my medicine?

Acupuncturists do not have the right to make recommendations about this. Patients can be told that it is often possible to decrease their medications but their symptoms must improve first (e.g. blood glucose levels in diabetics). They can be encouraged to monitor their progress, and to consult with their physicians regarding their current dosage and strength of medication. Cortisone, blood pressure medication and codeine are frequently the subject of questions about reducing dosages or discontinuing the medication when people are receiving TCM treatment.

Last time I didn't feel any pain, but today every needle feels painful.

Why is that?

Although you may use the same needling technique and the same group of points, sometimes a patient may experience different needling sensations from usual.

The likely explanation is that the meridians are opening and the patient's energy is just beginning to flow. This is a good sign that the body is responding and becoming more sensitive to treatment. Generally the patient's symptoms are improving at the same time, so do not worry about this increased sensitivity.

Another reason may be that a patient has arrived at your office right after rushing or exercising, so the energy is closer to the surface of the skin. This is still all right, but it is best to invite the person to relax for a while in your waiting area before beginning the treatment.

I have had one or two treatments, and now I feel like I am getting

worse. Why?

The effects of acupuncture are cumulative, so for some conditions it may take some time before acupuncture begins to produce measurable results, and the condition may appear to be still declining. More frequent treatments may be called for at this time, when a patient will finally see rapid improvement. This slump is called a 'healing crisis'. The body is complicated; sometimes we need to give a lengthy chance for therapies to work. We cannot expect a miracle every time. A healing crisis is more apt to occur in Bi syndromes and other painful conditions involving the extremities. Patients will find this occurrence less alarming if they have been warned about this possibility.

What can I do at home to help my condition?

Of course, a trained TCM practitioner will know what to suggest in terms of diet, exercise and other lifestyle changes to support a patient's health. But we sometimes need to spend time doing research and talking to more experienced practitioners in order to create a complete lifestyle programme for a patient with a life-threatening illness. Examples of conditions that may require this are kidney failure, severe diabetes, poststroke paralysis, cancer and severe heart and circulatory conditions. A complete lifestyle programme would include a diet suggesting certain vegetables and fruits, exercise like qigong or taiji, sleep, water intake and other activities such as meditation, support groups and creative outlets like music or artwork.

A regularly updated list of what services and classes are offered in the local community is a great practical tool for practitioner and patient alike. Patients who are feeling unwell may lack the energy to look for a qigong class, but might go if they know when and where these are held and whom to call for information. It is also extremely helpful to have handouts ready on exercise, nutrition, responses to grief, etc. that can be given to patients as needed; these should have the practitioner's name and contact information on them, which will help keep the practitioner in the patient's mind.

In follow-up appointments, the practitioner can ask the patient how the new programme is going, provide encouragement, and if necessary adjust the programme to make it more workable. Some people's willpower may be strong in the face of a serious illness; for others it is extremely difficult to make changes – a situation that calls for our compassion and understanding.

Questions patients don't ask

Some of the most important things patients need to know in order to benefit fully from treatment are questions they do not know enough to ask. These are issues practitioners often neglect to address. For instance, people who are new to acupuncture need to be taught how to prepare for treatment. If they have acupuncture when they are hungry, dehydrated or immediately after heavy physical activity, the energy flow may cause them to feel faint or nauseated.

Suggest that for at least a couple of hours after treatment it is best to avoid strenuous activity, a long drive or a late night, which may result in fatigue or feelings of illness. Sexual activity takes energy, so is also not recommended immediately after acupuncture. Patients should be told not to bathe within a few hours of acupuncture, because it will disturb the energy flow and there is a small possibility of infection. A short list of 'things you can do to get the most from your treatment' could easily be included on an information handout or brochure.

Also, teach patients that every treatment will be received differently, depending on a multitude of environmental, emotional and mental factors. Often benefits are felt during the days following a treatment rather than on the day of the treatment. Especially if you are doing a strong treatment with many needles, patients should be warned that they might feel significant fatigue or even mildly flu-like symptoms for a day or two; this is a sign that healing processes are occurring. Also acupuncture can take people out of 'overdrive' so that they really experience their true state of fatigue, if that is their underlying condition. If they don't know this, patients may think the practitioner has done something to make them feel worse.

LIFESTYLE EDUCATION

Traditionally, Chinese medicine is as much about maintaining health as it is about curing disease. A basic tenet of TCM is to encourage people to take responsibility for their own wellness. So we have a wonderful opportunity to help patients – and the community in which we practice – learn about and work with the many lifestyle and environmental factors that affect their long-term health.

It is up to acupuncturists to develop expertise in preventative areas of TCM in order to educate patients, to decide how much time and energy to dedicate to this aspect of their practice, and how best to go about doing so. One practical way is to create brochures with information about various aspects of Oriental medicine, its underlying philosophy, maintaining health and promoting healing with energy nourishing exercises like taiji and qigong. A rack of these in a clinic's waiting area is an information resource for patients and for other members of the community who want to find out more. Some acupuncturists have a list of recommended books or even a lending library available for those who want to explore the subject in depth.

Another way to educate the public is to present seminars, either at the acupuncture clinic if there is sufficient space, or at a local community centre, hall or church meeting room. This gives a forum for people to ask questions and to gain comfort with the acupuncturist as a person as well as receiving valuable health information. A series of seminars offered during the autumn or spring seasons can also be a rich educational experience.

In general, if acupuncturists practising in the West consider themselves as educators of a whole approach to well-being, they will prepare themselves as teachers to answer people's questions, to direct people to classes and to written material that will help them, and to model the balanced living promoted by Chinese medicine to the extent which they are able.

Nutrition

An old Chinese proverb says 'diseases enter into the body through the mouth'; in other words, most disorders are related to diet. Even if patients don't ask about this, it is always a good idea to offer them tips on affordable, accessible foods that will help their condition.

Nutritional education can be a challenge for a practitioner working in the West. Although many people are concerned about nutrition, there are many conflicting views on the proper way to eat. These days it is popular to eat raw food based on the idea that raw foods are richest in enzymes. Eating a certain way according to your blood type is another approach. North Americans in particular are seeking a cure for obesity by trying a variety of diets with varying levels of nutritional balance.

The question of how best they should nourish themselves is confusing and often overwhelming for people, especially when they are facing a health crisis. Providing nutritional information within the context of TCM can be very helpful for some patients. Raising awareness about the natures and temperatures of different foods, and the effects of the flavours, and tailoring this information for an individual's needs would be a great service to him or her.

Many practitioners find it works best when they write down for patients a list of available foods, and explain *why* these foods are selected according to TCM theory ('because this clears Heat, which is causing this symptom', for example). Patients need to be told how long and how often to eat a particular food, and whether they need to take a break from eating it. Give as much detail as possible regarding dietary changes.

Part of the practitioner's own education could include discovering the nearest and best local sources of Chinese herbs and healing foods, or if these are inaccessible, then Western herbal stores, or even where people can find good quality produce.

The acupuncturist could print up 'how to' sheets on preparing congees, or lists of easily available foods that support different organ systems, to pass out to suitable patients. A more ambitious educational effort, of benefit to the whole community, would be to present cooking classes based on TCM. Each class in a series could be focused on a different element or on how to build qi, blood, yin and so on.

Exercise

Everyone has heard that exercise benefits health yet, just like nutritional information, there are thousands of ways that are purported to be of benefit. Under the umbrella of TCM are age-old practices of energy-restoring exercises. An acupuncturist could teach people about the possibility of moving their bodies in nourishing, supportive ways. Perhaps it is beyond the scope of acupuncture practice actually to teach qigong or other similar forms of exercise, but to know who in your area does teach qigong or taiji and how people may get in contact with them would encourage people to explore this outside your clinic.

If this subject is especially interesting to you and you are studying a form of taiji or qigong, it is possible to form a group of keen people who meet and practise together bi-weekly or whatever schedule works for the group. Groups are often cherished by members for their capacity to support them in doing what they know is good for them but do not feel personally motivated to do alone. You may be able to find some local teachers, or good classes at the local recreation centre, that you can recommend to suitable patients. Qigong is extremely helpful for people undergoing medical treatment for cancer, to boost their energy and immune systems and help them withstand side-effects of treatment.

Emotional/spiritual education

In TCM, we emphasise that qi, essence and spirit are the three basic components of our health. The term 'spirit' is not necessarily related or restricted to its religious meaning, but in TCM can be used to cover thought, emotion and dream analysis. In our assessment of patients, it is as important to understand their spirit as it is to find a diagnosis and differentiation of syndromes. Peace of mind is inseparable from overall health.

Spiritual education often involves changing ways of thinking, viewing, experiencing and reacting to things happening in the living environment from the point of view of what is good for health. It is only when we address people's minds that qi can move more freely through the body, and will respond to the acupuncture treatment much more quickly and strongly.

Since many energy imbalances originate in part in unresolved emotional issues or living in conditions of stress, it would be wise for acupuncturists to actively teach emotional well-being. Living in our modern fast-paced world often means that we have little time for reflection and digestion of the daily tumults that occur. Simply teaching about pausing throughout the day, like a miniature meditation moment, can be enormously helpful for some people.

One of the philosophical gifts of TCM is its non-judgmental approach to emotions. Emotions are 'energy in motion', qi flowing in specific directions and associated with specific organ systems. This concept is neutral and allows people to step back and witness their emotional energy with more compassion.

Meditation is one of the foundations of balanced living according to many forms of traditional medicine. Instructing patients how to meditate or directing them to meditation teachers or groups in the area is well worth considering as part of your holistic service.

Family support

Spouse and family support and participation can make a huge difference to a patient trying to change life patterns. Because of the time-consuming nature and far-reaching impacts of a lifestyle program, you may plan a special appointment with the patient *and* the family in order to introduce it to them. You could then explain the reasons for your recommendations, and elicit the family's support in food preparation, shopping, phoning and driving to appointments, etc. All this takes time and energy, but is of great benefit to the patient, who will do better with active family support.

DEALING WITH DIFFICULT PATIENTS
Challenging or intractable cases

If, after six or eight treatments in the space of one month or so, a patient has experienced no significant improvement, or perhaps a worsening of symptoms, this is a challenging case. This calls for extra thought and effort on the part of the practitioner. Analyse each treatment – which symptoms are better and which are worse – and clarify which organ systems are mainly involved. Have you focused enough attention on those systems? Ask yourself if you have made the correct diagnosis, and are therefore heading in the right direction. Are your treatments strong enough, or stimulating enough? If employing other therapeutic modalities such as herbs, are they the proper herbs to use in this case and, if so, have you designed the correct combination? Be careful about what condition patients say they have and what they really have; often they are just guessing.

Make a chart to pay close attention to all the factors affecting the person's experience, including stress, lifestyle changes, diet, medications, weather changes, menstrual cycle, and time of day that symptoms worsen. Sometimes patients with migraines, for example, will chart their lives at home and work or school, providing you with a treasury of clues about what's causing the headaches.

After gleaning what information you can about similar cases by consulting books, journals and the internet, and talking to other practitioners, you will be ready to make a new treatment plan. Before implementing this plan, give your patient 1 to 2 weeks off in order to break the established cycle and to begin afresh.

Follow the new treatment plan for one or two courses of six to eight treatments apiece, noting all the while whether it seems to be effective. If, after this, the results are still not as desired, it is time to refer the patient to a senior practitioner in the area. It may also be advisable to re-consult with the patient's physician. Develop a list of other TCM practitioners or other health care providers you are comfortable referring to.

If the nearest experienced TCM practitioner is some distance away, you could accompany your patient, and learn during or after the treatment how better to diagnose and treat him or her. Once this difficult situation has been resolved, the patient may still find it most convenient to continue to see you in your office.

Emotionally complex patients

No one working in the health field can entirely avoid meeting emotionally challenging patients. Every practitioner will encounter this situation at one time or another. Learning how to care for difficult patients effectively will help your practice run smoothly with fewer problems.

In general there are two types of challenging patients. The first includes those who have a lot of experience with many health practitioners of all fields, and who criticise everything from your treatment style to the paint colour in your room. These people arrive ready to doubt your ability to help them. The other type of difficult patient has serious health concerns, and will also project on to you their emotional confusion, sadness, anger and impatience.

Difficult patients commonly exhibit some of the following characteristics:

- asking many challenging questions during the first visit, for example, 'Why don't you have the equipment that Dr So-and-so has?'
- after the first treatment, adding complicating symptoms and claiming that these were caused by or related to your first treatment
- showing a generally unfriendly and tense attitude
- after their major concern improves or is cured, they dismiss its importance and suddenly complain of a big new concern that they then try to link with the first problem; for example, a woman with knee pain which quickly improves then complains of thigh pain and attributes its cause to the treatment for the knee.

One can make extra efforts to make someone like this happy. However, be aware that such people are often unhappy and dissatisfied with their lives, and therefore try to make others take responsibility for them. These patients present obstacles the acupuncturist will need to learn how to negotiate around smoothly in order to help them as much as possible, and for the practitioner's professional relationship with them to reach a satisfactory conclusion. When dealing with difficult patients, it is especially important to chart everything in detail.

The first step is to recognise and accept that this is an emotionally difficult patient. The practitioner needs to be prepared psychologically to have compassion and not to take the patient's attitude too personally. Anticipate that it will take more time than usual to communicate with them, for example, scheduling their appointment at the end of the day or on the weekend. Understand that, besides their health concern, they may have family problems, trouble in relationships or financial stress, all of which contribute to their sadness, impatience or frustration.

When treating emotionally difficult people, it is advisable to take small steps: using fewer needles, retaining needles for a shorter period of time and minimising stimulation. Making greater use of therapeutic methods like tui na or acupressure will help obtain results with less stress. Use caution with all methods. Use herbs carefully, combining those with gentler functions to begin with. This gentle approach can help to avoid strong reactions, as even positive changes can feel overwhelming to some people.

Ask for advice from more experienced practitioners. If both the senior practitioner and the patient agree, send this patient to the senior practitioner for a couple of visits for some new ideas on diagnosis and treatment.

Arrange your treatment plan carefully, allowing for a break of 2 weeks to 1 month after the course of treatment decided upon is complete. Sometimes when you resume treatments a softer energy will be evident in the person, owing to a shift in family situation, improved relationships with friends, a holiday or a job change. This is an important principle to learn as a practitioner. Sometimes active treatments promote healing, and sometimes no action heals. This is the Taoist idea of wu wei or 'action without doing'. This means that you may need to be patient and not try to push the treatment too quickly in the direction you think it should go. The situation may resolve itself naturally.

Although someone may complain continually and challenge you excessively, they may still want to receive treatment from you, even when you suggest that they see someone else or take a break from treatment. Another option would be to invite a second practitioner with much life experience, preferably of the same sex as the patient, to treat the patient together with you for at least a couple of visits. This may provide protection for you in that the second practitioner can be a witness to the situation. It also may make the patient feel specially taken care of, which could ease the pattern of relating that you have had to date. Of course, before taking this action you will have had sufficient conversation with the second practitioner, and have obtained consent from the patient.

In some instances, you could mention the benefits that may be derived from counselling, and even offer the name of a professional counsellor you know and trust. Of course it is up to the patient to choose to follow this suggestion or not.

If none of the above suggestions is effective, there is always the option of handing over the patient to another practitioner. Referring is not letting someone down, but helping the person to receive help from someone whose skills or personality may offer a better fit. A confidential conversation with the new practitioner about the way in which he or she is approaching the case is likely to add to your knowledge of how to deal with a similarly challenging patient in the future.

Also, be open to the possibility that difficult patients may be triggering some of your own emotional issues. Someone, for instance, may remind you of your own controlling parent – a manifestation that in psychological terms is called countertransference. Practitioners can learn a great deal from these patients if we take the time to listen and reflect.

References

Zhu, Hong Zhen 2003 Building a jade screen: better health with Chinese medicine. Penguin, Toronto; first published by Prentice Hall, Scarborough, Ontario, 2001

Professional development and clinic management

INTRODUCTION

As health professionals, most of our attention is appropriately given to the proper care of our patients. However, the most caring and skilled acupuncturists may be unable to run a successful practice if they lack basic management skills. Sadly, many excellent practitioners have abandoned our profession because they could not make a living. Perhaps they were setting up in an area where there is already too much competition, or they didn't know how to attract potential patients. A successful acupuncturist resists complacency, and instead continues to refine and deepen technique, and gain knowledge.

Good clinic management is important not just to the practitioner's livelihood but also to the patients' well-being. Slovenly habits in the clinic and poor record keeping may, at minimum, cause patients to lose confidence in an acupuncturist's professional abilities. More seriously, they can lead to treatment errors and even injuries.

Styles of practice vary widely from country to country and practitioner to practitioner, so this book does not pretend to be the definitive guide. I simply offer some points, gathered from my own experience and suggestions from several respected colleagues, which you may find helpful to consider as you set up and run your own practice.

Developing skills in treatment planning

8

The skilled acupuncturist knows how to keep an eye on today's treatment while maintaining a longer view of helping the patient get well. During the first few visits, the practitioner gradually forms an idea of the disease pattern exhibited by this patient, how it should be treated, how often, for how long, and what kind of changes can be expected.

Knowing the general nature of many patterns and how these behave with treatment is only one part of the story. Equally important is the individual nature of this particular patient. Individual patients will have their own special features – age, constitution, level of sensitivity to certain treatments or points, etc. that need to be taken into account. Theoretical knowledge combined with a detailed understanding of each patient's needs creates the whole picture, which is called the treatment plan.

It generally only takes one or two sessions to get an idea of how a particular patient is responding to treatment. This tells us whether the patient's problem is likely to be resolved after another couple of treatments, whether the person needs to come more or less frequently for a longer period of time, or whether help is needed that the acupuncturist cannot give. As always, the decision is based on the best interest of the patient, and not on the practitioner's desire to effect a 'cure' no matter how long it takes.

INITIAL EVALUATION

During the first consultation with a patient, it is important to determine the seriousness of the case. If a patient's activity and daily functioning are being limited significantly, a symptom can be deemed as serious. Even if a patient's original complaints seem relatively minor, there are likely to be other indications that the person may be susceptible to a chronic condition. A detailed patient intake form is a useful tool (see the section on effective record keeping for more information about these) and can include a 'SUDS' (subjective units of distress) assessment. On a scale of 1–10, how does the patient rate the seriousness of the symptom?

Clinical observations such as the colour and texture of the skin, clearness in the eyes and condition of the tongue would also offer clues. More subtle indications might be the degree of frankness the patient exhibits about symptoms, openness of expression, the posture of the patient, or the ability to make human contact. As a result, despite the fact that the patient may come in with a common complaint, further discussion may reveal deeper anxieties, recurring depressions or low self-esteem. In these cases, where progress may not be quick or easy, the patient should be told to expect some difficulties and have patience. Such a case may present many problems during the process of healing, and the end result may not even be a definite cure.

In situations where a person's life may be threatened or the quality of life severely limited, it is crucial to understand the significance of a particular symptom. Only then is it possible for you to have confidence in your chosen treatment and a clear awareness of the boundaries of your expertise. When you recognise the limitations of TCM in general and your own skills in particular, when faced with a set of symptoms you don't know how to deal with, it becomes much easier to determine whether or when to refer the patient to another practitioner, to a different kind of practitioner, or to a hospital. Whether you refer patients to a physician or an alternative practitioner, do not forget to discuss the issues carefully with the patient who has come to you to seek help.

After making a decision as to the seriousness of the case, the next task is to determine the correct remedy. For inexperienced practitioners, this decision can be quite difficult, especially when faced with chronic cases. However, it is a decision that should not be made without taking great care. The first remedy is the one that opens up the case, setting it either in a direction toward true healing or toward confusion and disorder.

Sometimes, the initial case is quite evident. The patient speaks of a few routine complaints; you immediately see a clear fit with a particular treatment plan and will feel confidence in proceeding with it. Even though you may be relatively inexperienced, you will see results when the initial diagnosis is clear and obvious.

The more common situation, however, is a mixture of symptom pictures. For example, a patient may present symptoms such as a headache, red face and short temper, and you will naturally think this person has an upsurge of Liver fire. But upon more questioning, it turns out that this person actually has more Liver and Kidney yin deficiency symptoms. After more thought and study, it will turn out that the patient is suffering from Liver yang rising. This pattern is different from that of an upsurge of Liver fire. The latter exhibits excess Heat in both symptoms and root, whereas in Liver yang rising, symptoms look like excess but the root is yin deficiency.

It can take some work to design a treatment plan that actually covers the entirety of the symptoms. Not every symptom may be dealt with, but one hopes to design a treatment that clearly covers the majority of the most important symptoms, as well as addressing the underlying cause.

DESIGNING A TREATMENT PLAN

Generally speaking, patients fall into one of these categories: acute, chronic, or maintenance. People move between these as their conditions change, but the practitioner should know to which category any individual patient belongs at the time of each visit. This awareness directs treatment planning.

A treatment plan covers:

- the diagnosis based on all information gathered from history, interview, tongue picture, pulses and palpation
- the treatment principle
- acupuncture point selection, combinations and other treatment modalities
- an outline of the expected course of treatment, indicating the commitment of time and money.

Acute cases usually need between one and eight treatments to resolve the problem. A treatment every other day over 1 to 2 weeks may be necessary. Some conditions that may require this approach are acute muscle injury, severe sciatica, shingles in the acute phase, acute Bell's palsy, acute arthritis pain and swelling, including rheumatoid, colds, flu and severe cough.

For chronic cases, the acupuncturist will usually see a person for a few courses of treatment. A course generally comprises six to ten treatments, or one to two treatments per week for 1 to 3 months. Intervals between treatment courses are normally 1 to 2 weeks. Conditions that fall into this category include: chronic lower back pain, chronic intestinal conditions such as irritable bowel syndrome or colitis, frozen shoulder, tennis elbow, tendonitis, heartburn, menopausal symptoms, anxiety, depression, chronic fatigue, poststroke syndrome, infertility and many TCM zang-fu disorders.

As we know, acupuncture effects are generally cumulative; in other words each treatment adds to the effects of previous treatments. However, if the same groups of acupuncture points are used repeatedly, the body's response to them will diminish. The rate of improvement will naturally slow and the treatment becomes less effective. One way to avoid this plateau is to alternate, visit to visit, between two groups of acupuncture points. Each group has major and supplementary points; the major ones are used almost every time while the supplementary points change at each treatment. Another way to break through a plateau is to take a 2–4 week break from treatments. When treatment resumes, the body will have a fresh response.

Maintenance conditions usually call for treatment only once a week to once per month, or even less frequently. Examples of this are deficient wei qi or weak immune system, general qi and blood deficiency, sleep disturbance from stress, zang-fu disharmony such as hyperactive Liver yang, and hormonal disruptions associated with menopause or thyroid imbalance. Some people only need a seasonal 'tune-up' for their allergies, asthma or seasonal affective disorder – the winter 'blues'.

Many patients come in with multiple complaints rather than a single concern that could be set right quickly. One way to proceed is to treat first the problem that is 'speaking the loudest' – in other words the most acute. If the primary complaint is not causing the patient major discomfort, it could be left until the more easily resolved issues have been addressed. This gives both practitioner and patient the satisfaction of having already achieved some treatment goals.

SCHEDULING

Balancing the needs of patients and practitioners

Many new practitioners find that allowing 1 to 1½ hours for each patient is not only less stressful for the acupuncturist, but gives enough time for a thorough history, accurate and detailed diagnosis and a relaxed treatment. Even when a practitioner develops enough experience and efficiency to tighten the schedule, it is advisable to book 1½ hours for first-time patients, or even 2 hours if the initial phone conversation with a patient suggests the case is extraordinary or complicated. After a few sessions with some patients, it may become evident that they need a longer treatment time for cupping, tui na, etc.

Scheduling a 5–10 minute break between patients gives practitioners time to wash their hands, prepare the treatment table and look at notes for the next patient without falling behind in the day's schedule.

Scheduling a mixture of new and long-term patients in a half or whole day helps keep the acupuncturist's mind fresh. Also, avoid booking two complicated cases in a row if possible. If one of them is scheduled at the end of the day, there is more time to spend with the patient.

Acupuncturists in their first few months of practice, especially those who have no receptionist in the clinic, usually find it best not to book full days.

Time is needed during the day to keep up with paperwork, study and – one hopes – answering calls from people who want to make an appointment.

Another suggestion for new practitioners: even if you are not very busy at first, try to be available for several hours every day rather than for only a couple of full days a week. Over the years, I have observed that new practitioners who are accessible for only a couple of days a week tend to have more trouble attracting patients than those who are in the clinic every day, even if it is just for a few hours. Keeping daily office hours also makes it easier to answer telephone messages promptly. People with health problems generally expect to have their calls returned within 24 hours; otherwise they may feel that the clinic has no interest in them.

Some practitioners choose to telephone appointment reminders to patients who are very busy or who tend to be absentminded. Patients are more likely to turn up to appointments if they are given a card that has the acupuncturist's name, address and telephone number, and a space for three or four appointment dates and times.

Last-minute cancellations are a major annoyance, and new practitioners are frequently unsure of how to handle the issue of whether or not to charge patients for missed appointments. Some practitioners give a one-time grace to patients; everyone forgets an appointment at one time or another and if a patient doesn't make a habit of this it is nice to be understanding about an occasional memory lapse. If someone cancels at short notice because of a personal or family emergency, or can't get to your office because of a storm, blocked road or dead battery, there's not much one can do beyond take a deep breath, enjoy the break and perhaps practise a little qigong! That's life.

If patients call at the last minute to cancel because they have developed a headache that may actually be related to the complaint, you may gently suggest that a treatment will help both the new symptom and the underlying cause, though of course you should not insist. If the patient chooses not to come in, it is a judgement call as to whether to bill for this appointment.

However, when a person cancels at short notice or simply fails to turn up without a good reason, or is a habitual no-show, most practitioners will expect payment anyway. Your policy on this can and should be posted in the clinic, may be included on your telephone-answering message, and can be written on the back of your card with a line like: 'This appointment time has been reserved for you. Please give at least 24 hours notice if you cannot keep this time.' If you wish to take a harder line on this, you can even indicate that patients will be billed for missed appointments.

Treatment timing for better results

Some patients like to get all their medical appointments over with in one day, and will call to arrange an acupuncture treatment after they've booked appointments with their chiropractor, dentist or physiotherapist. It is best to discourage patients from doing this, as their body can become overstimulated and exhausted. Obviously this is counterproductive for obtaining a good treatment result. Another reason it is inadvisable to schedule many appointments on the same day is that, if the patient has an adverse reaction, it would be difficult to distinguish the cause of it.

There are some conditions in which the timing of the treatment influences how effective it will be. Here are a few examples:

Timing of treatment according to condition

—For dysmenorrhoea, irregular menstruation or PMS related to Liver qi stagnation, it is best to treat 5 to 7 days before the onset of menses (according to the woman's cycle over the previous 2 months). If the symptoms are the result of Kidney deficiency, timing is not so crucial; treatment can be given right after the period, or even 7–10 days later.
—For insomnia or frequent nocturia, afternoon and early evening treatments are better than those earlier in the day, because the treatment effects take a few hours to set in. Once that happens, the person is ready to sleep.
—For working on hypertension or digestive disorders such as irritable bowel syndrome, gastric reflux or bloating after meals, morning treatments are better than those in the afternoon, because the patient should have a number of waking hours available for eating, drinking and activities that encourage good bowel movement. The patient does not want to have to wake up in the night for it. In addition, each treatment imprints the brain with the suggestion that the bowel movement occurs at the same time every day.

These are just a few of many cases in which the factor of treatment timing needs to be taken into account when booking patients.

Scheduling breaks in courses of treatment

When patients reach a certain level of improvement or cure, it is time to let them go. Here we are not talking about long-term patients who come in for a seasonal tune-up a couple of times a year, or who come in for an immune booster during flu season, or are experiencing extra stress; it refers to continuing to treat someone whose condition has pretty much cleared up.

Releasing patients keeps the patient load cycling or flowing through the practice and opens up space for new patients. Not all practitioners will agree with this view, but letting patients go, when you have done as much as you can for them, gives them the satisfying sense that they have reached a goal.

Ethically speaking, it is not healthy to allow a patient to create a dependence on a practitioner, or to hang on to someone forever unless it is palliative care.

When treating acute conditions, the right time to stop treatment is usually obvious: the condition is resolved or vastly improved. It is less obvious with chronic or recurring illnesses, but a general guideline is when a group of symptoms quietens, or when an intermittent condition does not return for a significant period of time, perhaps 2 months.

At some point during the course of treatment, the acupuncturist will be able to anticipate how many more sessions seem appropriate before it is time to stop, and to indicate this in the treatment plan at least two or three visits in advance. At that stage it is appropriate to have a discussion with the patient about your rationale for taking a break.

Patients who are being released can be offered advice about supportive lifestyle measures such as diet and exercise, as well as an assurance that they are welcome to return if symptoms recur, or simply for a check-up and preventive treatment at some time in the future.

Single or group treatment

A decision about whether to see one patient or several at a time greatly depends on local cultural practices and to some degree the practitioner's own values. In China, for instance, because of the huge population and crowding, individual appointments are nearly impossible to obtain, and people are accustomed to conducting more of their private business in public. In Western countries seeing only one patient at a time may be detrimental to the practitioner's cash flow. However, patients may feel a lack of privacy if they are talking to their acupuncturist about symptoms or being treated while a total stranger is lying 1 metre away on the other side of a curtain. Even practitioners who prefer to focus their attention on one patient at a time sometimes will agree to overlap treatment times for family members or close friends if they are comfortable with this.

An acupuncturist who is running several treatment rooms must absolutely ensure that the patient who is being left while the next is being treated is warm, comfortable and not in pain. A patient left alone too long may feel nervous or neglected, and if experiencing an emotional release in response to the treatment may need the practitioner's caring attention.

Patients may also need to ask questions that come up during treatment. Believe it or not, there have been cases in which a patient with needles in has been forgotten, lying in a room for several hours.

EFFECTIVE RECORD KEEPING

Good records are an important tool in treatment planning. Even the simplest impromptu treatments should be noted. Records help set the future direction for treating each patient. They provide valuable information to study, analyse and improve the practitioner's knowledge and skills. And finally, records are required documents for legal investigations should they occur, and are protection for the practitioner if any questions are later raised about negligence or malpractice.

It is recommended that two types of record forms be used: a first visit or patient intake questionnaire, and a form for subsequent visits. The one for new patients is by far the most detailed and thorough, which will ensure that nothing important is missed regarding the person's health, history or current concerns. It should include the following features:

Record forms

—Basic personal information such as name, address, phone number and profession. Consider including the patient's postal code (for writing if the clinic relocates), treatment time of day (a.m./p.m.) and where the patient heard about you. This last question elicits useful information about where word-of-mouth advertising is coming from, which helps develop ways to make the practice known in the community
—Information such as the patient's age may sometimes be asked for indirectly, for example, by asking how old the person was when an accident occurred, and how many years have elapsed since then
—Chief complaint and the history of this illness, not only how long the person has had symptoms, but also if there has been a Western medical diagnosis, how long ago and what treatment is being or has been undergone
—Family history of serious conditions such as heart disease, cancer, diabetes, or lifestyle and environmental issues (working environment, or having grown up in a polluted area)
—Any medications or supplements being taken
—Any allergies to medication
—Any previous acupuncture treatments, and the patient's response; this helps ascertain whether the person has had unusual reactions such as extreme sensitivity, fainting, etc.
—A questionnaire/checklist covering the basic questions necessary for TCM diagnosis, such as chills and fever, headache, body pain, urine, stool, sweat, chest, abdomen, period and pregnancy for women, immunisation for children and so on
—The practitioner's notes based on the patient interview: assessment, diagnosis, prediction of progress, course and steps of treatment and expectations of results.

Notes should also include tongue picture, pulses, TCM diagnosis and treatment principle and plan, as well as point selection and the technique used for each point. The order in which points are recorded may not be the same as the order in which needles are inserted, owing to the patient's position or other factors. A logical way to do this is to record the main points first, and separated by a space, record the supplementary points. Each group of points may be recorded in the order of: (a) upper body to lower body, (b) front of the body to the back, (c) medial to lateral or (d) head and trunk to limbs and extremities.

Include, in addition, all treatment modalities given such as herbs, moxibustion, cupping, tui na (name meridian or area) and lifestyle recommendations. If raw herbs or patent medicines have been prescribed, record the dosage (number of grams or number of pills) and prescribed use (number of times per day). This is important information to have if the patient later experiences ill effects. Also record the patient's position on the treatment table since, depending on results, this may influence subsequent treatment choices.

Lastly, it is crucial to immediately write down what happens during the actual treatment (i.e. the patient's responses and reactions to certain acupoints and techniques). For example, note whether a patient feels particularly tender or nervous at a specific point, and the reason. Perhaps there is scar tissue there. One patient I treated did not like electrical stimulation because it reminded her of a single childhood seizure she once had. Record the other extreme too, when a patient loves a certain point, such as Yin Tang, because she feels calm, focused and happy when this point is needled.

Before each visit, it is a good idea to refresh one's memory of the patient by reviewing notes of the last few treatments. If this is a difficult case, a well-prepared practitioner will have analysed the patient's condition after the previous visit, and designed a treatment plan for this session.

For most regular patients, writing records is done during the treatment, especially notes on patients' reactions to certain points and techniques, and is finished up between patients or at the end of the day. For complicated cases, it helps to write rough notes immediately and a good copy after conducting some research later that day or the following day.

Sometimes simple pictures are very helpful in records, in order to show the areas of pain or disorder on a patient's body. Shading can be used to indicate these areas.

Refining needling technique and diagnostic skills

9

However excellent an acupuncturist's formal training has been, refining diagnostic and technical skills is a lifelong process. For the first several months of practice, a tremendous amount can be learned by sitting down at the end of each day and analysing treatments. What worked today? What did not work today, or why did a patient feel pain today? It could be that the person was experiencing premenstrual syndrome, depression or had had a particularly trying week. It could be that you were too nervous or stiff, or used a new order of imperfect needles. (If you suspect the latter case, check needle tips with a magnifying glass to see whether they are rough or hooked, or brush the tips with a cotton ball to see if any fibres catch.)

In any medical discipline, we learn it is sometimes necessary to cause a patient discomfort in order to work toward a cure. But there are ways to minimise this discomfort without compromising the effectiveness of treatment; these methods are not always taught in acupuncture schools.

When you practise your needling technique, warm up your joints first so that your hand becomes flexible, loose and decisive. This way you will show new patients, whose major concern is pain, that your technique is mature enough, especially as they are particularly primed to be nervous with a new practitioner. Therefore, the first several needles inserted painlessly are crucial to build trust with a patient.

ANALYSIS AND PREVENTION OF PAIN IN ACUPUNCTURE

In acupuncture, pain can result on inserting the needle, on withdrawing it or after the treatment. When a needle stimulates receptors in nerves, blood vessels, muscles or most other tissues it will cause pain. But the pain threshold varies from person to person, and the level of discomfort experienced differs in various locations. For instance, in thin muscle, such as the face and the fingers and toes, a needle insertion will always be uncomfortable, if not painful.

The cuticular layer of the skin is full of nerve endings, capillaries and many pain receptors, which are likely to respond with a sharp sensation when a needle goes in. But when the needle is inserted quickly enough to get through this layer and into the subcutaneous layer, the sensation of pain will be briefer and less acute.

Usually, a properly placed needle rests in muscle and soft tissue, causing sensations of aching and distension. This is the way de qi, or the arrival of qi, is most frequently experienced.

The patient's different sensations are clues to what kind of tissue is underneath the needle, and whether its insertion is correct or needs slight alteration.

It is worth reiterating here that I am talking about the levels of discomfort that may arise from the normal insertion of needles by a properly trained and competent acupuncturist, and not the kind of errors in depth and angle that cause injuries such as those examined in detail in Section One.

That said, if the patient feels a severe sharp pain when a needle is placed below the skin, a small blood vessel has probably been pricked. If the needle is already in and the patient suddenly experiences a sharp pain, it is usually because the person has moved, slightly dislodging the needle so that it is touching a nerve or blood vessel. In either case, the needle should be withdrawn slightly, the angle changed, and the needle returned to the correct depth. Wait 2–3 seconds before adjusting the angle. If the new angle is still causing pain, then the needle has to be removed and replaced 1–2 mm from the initial site.

When a needle touches a tendon, ligament, or the periosteum covering a bone, it normally causes a bearable aching, soreness and occasionally heaviness. This is fine, again as long as the needle simply nears or touches the surface of these tissues but does not penetrate them. However, if insertion has been too aggressive, driving the needle tip into these tougher tissues, the needle tip can bend, causing severe pain when the needle is stimulated. The way to distinguish this kind of pain from others is to listen to what the needle is telling you: when it is rotated, it will feel as though it has edges rather than being round (Fig. 9.1). The only correct way to proceed is to remove this needle and replace it more carefully.

Pain on removal of a needle at the end of the treatment is normally the result of one of two factors: either the patient is nervous or cold, which has contracted their muscles, or the rotation of the needle in one direction during the treatment has caused muscle fibres to twine around and grip the needle (Fig. 9.2). Yanking it straight out will mean severe discomfort for the patient. If the needle has been turned clockwise during treatment, first rotate it slightly in the opposite direction before removing it. Secondly, use the tips of the fingers to tap the muscles surrounding the point to relax the muscles and allow the needle to be more easily withdrawn. For more suggestions on releasing a stuck needle, refer to the section on carelessness with needles in Section One.

Pain after treatment is most often caused by the needle having injured a small vessel or punctured a nerve ending while it was being inserted, during treatment or on withdrawal. This may result in bruising or a small haematoma, which is likely to be uncomfortable for the patient. If blood emerges with the needle, the injury will normally result in a bruise. Gentle pressure on the site will help prevent blood from pooling under the skin. The patient should be reassured that any discomfort or bruising will disappear after a couple of days. Bruising, its prevention and treatment are also covered in more detail in Section One.

Figure 9.1 When a needle feels as though it has 'edges' while it is being rotated, its tip has probably been bent.

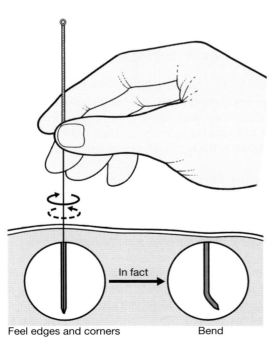

Feel edges and corners   Bend

Figure 9.2 Muscle fibres entwined around a needle.

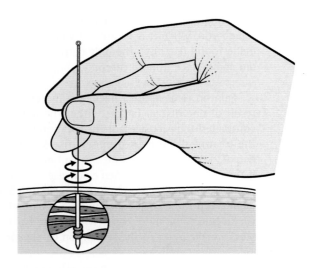

It sometimes happens that a patient will feel an aching or tingling in an arm or leg after treatment. This is a normal reaction to treatment as energy is moving around, and should disappear after 4 or 5 hours. The patient may need to be advised that it is best to avoid overexertion until the aching goes away. If the patient experiences such sensations whenever acupuncture is done on that arm or leg, it is a signal to the practitioner to reduce the amount and intensity of needle stimulation during this person's treatment.

TECHNIQUES FOR LESS PAINFUL NEEDLE INSERTION AND REMOVAL

Needle insertion in textbooks addresses the use of both hands, cotton balls and how to hold the skin, but often neglects the critical act of puncturing the skin with as little discomfort to the patient as possible.

Speed and accuracy are the key! If a needle's placement is too shallow, its tip will be probing the sensory nerves under the skin – and causing pain. But if it can be placed at exactly the right point and depth quickly, the needle is in before the nerves have time to register and transmit pain signals. During this faster insertion, the hand that is not putting in the needle also has a role to play.

Use the thumb and index finger to stretch the skin tightly to 'fix' the point (Fig. 9.3). At the exact moment the needle is going in, press down with the thumb and finger; this technique distributes the sensation of pressure across a wider area, reducing pain (Fig. 9.4). This is the method most textbooks recommend for use on thicker tissues such as the back and abdomen.

The following two techniques are less commonly discussed. One involves using the thumbnail of the practitioner's opposite hand to press firmly, precisely on the acupoint for 3 seconds (Fig. 9.5). As you are removing your nail, pop the needle in quickly to the desired depth.

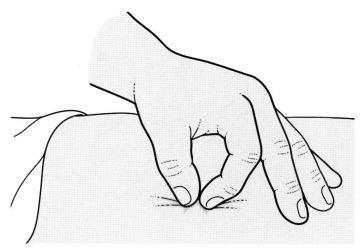

Figure 9.3 'Fixing' the acupoint.

The nerves cannot process two overlapping sensations – thumbnail pressure and needle pain – so the patient will feel a dull ache instead of a sharp pain.

The next technique is good for many points that tend to be sensitive, and is usually done with the shorter needles. The insertion is a controlled spinning throw, as of a rotating dart hitting the mark (Fig. 9.6). The distance of the throw is only around 0.5–1 cm, and the needle penetrates just past the nerve layer and into the subcutaneous tissue. The smaller distance offers more

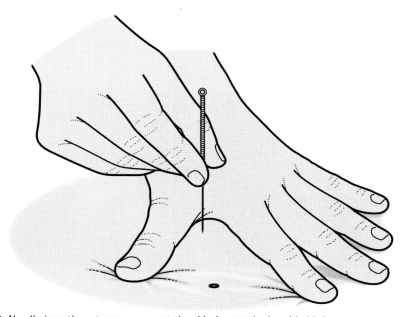

Figure 9.4 Needle insertion at same moment the skin is stretched and held down.

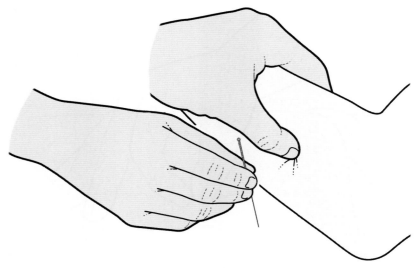

Figure 9.5 Thumbnail pressure obscures needle pain.

precision so is best used in sensitive areas, such as around the eyes and on the forehead. On limbs or the trunk, the larger throwing distance can be used.

Speed is also essential. This technique elicits a mild achy sensation, or no feeling at all. When you have a little bit more room to work in, you can use the thumb and index finger of your opposite hand to stretch and fix the skin around the acupoint.

Individual patients may also have uncomfortably sensitive or tender areas on their bodies where they prefer not be touched. On such a person, the

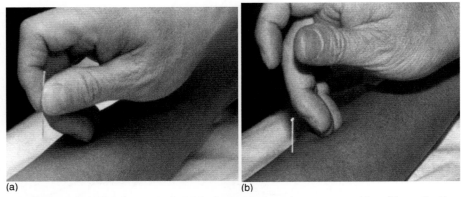

(a)   (b)

Figure 9.6a and b Acupuncturist 'spinning' a needle into the correct position. (Normally, the finger and thumb of opposite hand would be used to fix the skin, but have been left out of photo for the sake of visibility.)

acupuncturist may need to find a way to locate and needle this point without palpating it beforehand.

When a needle goes into a hair follicle (Fig. 9.7), it can be very painful; the tissue is very tight so trying to push it deeper just makes the pain worse. Withdraw the needle immediately, discard and replace with a new needle, being careful to avoid the follicle.

When treating back shu points on the Bladder meridians, needles are always put in at an oblique angle to avoid puncturing organs. But if the practitioner can feel the needle under the patient's skin, placement is too shallow – which will probably also be evident from the patient's complaints of sharp pain (Fig. 9.8). Back the needle off and adjust the angle on reinsertion

The tissue of the back is tougher and denser than other parts of the body, so the needle may actually bend underneath the skin causing severe pain. Tube needles are more likely to bend than the tubeless variety when they are being used on back points on the Bladder meridian.

To ensure needles are going into a back point at the correct angle, put the index finger of your other hand on the patient's skin when you make the insertion, so that you can feel it if the needle is bending. If you feel nothing, all is well.

When needling Ex. Ba Feng and Ex. Ba Xie points between the fingers and toes, it is less painful if needles are inserted as closely as possible to the web of skin, rather than toward the hand or foot.

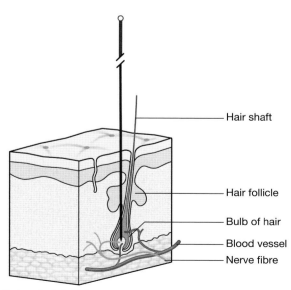

Hair shaft

Hair follicle

Bulb of hair

Blood vessel

Nerve fibre

Figure 9.7 A needle in a hair follicle.

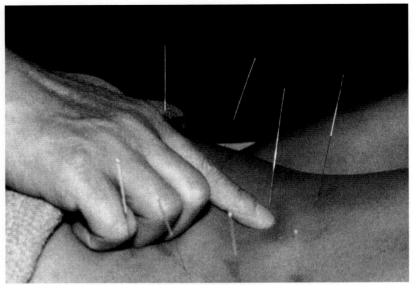

Figure 9.8 A practitioner checks the back shu points to ensure needle placement is not too shallow.

It is important to choose the right needle for the job. Needles that are too soft will bend too much on the way in and cause discomfort. Choose good quality needles that are firm but flexible. There are many brands of needles available; some are better than others.

Always be sure to remove a needle at the same angle and direction that it went in. Otherwise, the needle will dig into the tissues. When removing needles from a sensitive point, using a cotton ball to press on the point for a few seconds will always reduce pain.

Most common sensitive acupoints

Some points always elicit strong needle sensation and most people will feel some reaction such as an ache, tingling or nervousness when they are used. The most common examples are :

- LU-10
- LI-4, LI-11, LI-20
- SP-3, SP-4, SP-9
- HT-7
- SI-3
- BL-1

- KI-3
- PC-6
- TB-17
- LIV-3
- Du-26:

When treating a person who has never had acupuncture before, especially one who is worried about pain, it helps to avoid needling points you know will be particularly bad on the first visit. These can be massaged instead, or other points that share the same function but are less sensitive can be chosen. The patient will probably be able to relax more on a subsequent visit and accept a bit more discomfort.

One of my long-term patients provides an example of how a practitioner is regularly called upon to work with an individual's sensitivities. She has lots of body pain, a chronic sore throat and chronic Liver yang rising. Her final treatment points, LIV-3 and LU-10 are always sensitive, and can be uncomfortable to the degree that the entire treatment's energy flow is disturbed. When treating this woman, I always have to remember that pressing my fingernail into these points for 30 seconds to start the energy flow, and then quickly needling while she still feels the pressing sensation, eliminates her discomfort.

Needles with and without tubes

Some practitioners like to use needles with tubes because insertion is fast. They believe the speed of insertion will lessen the patient's pain. That is mostly true, but not always. The problem is that the needle can only penetrate the tissue to the depth the tube allows. That is fine for some points, but in others this predetermined depth is either too deep or too shallow. Most often, it is too shallow, leaving the tip of the needle lodged among sensory nerves. Then the acupuncturist has to readjust the needles manually. In my experience, patients report more pain when tube needles are used.

A new practitioner who always uses tube needles is at risk of losing technique in manual insertion, but it is reasonable to suggest that an intern use them for a period of time as he becomes more comfortable with needling, and his hand insertion technique develops.

Tube needles are useful in some situations: on points which experience has revealed are particularly sensitive, and on patients, especially children, whose fear of needles makes speedy insertion essential. Even in these situations, there are points where the use of tube needles is never appropriate, for instance where there is a small margin for error in depth, which could result in the puncture of a nerve or blood vessel.

A few practitioners use the acupuncture equivalent of a nail gun to shoot needles into the patient. This is not only painful, but also potentially dangerous; if a needle punctures the wall of the pleural cavity, air can be introduced, causing the lung to collapse. A manual insertion helps the acupuncturist sense the needle dropping into empty space – like putting a foot through the ceiling of the room below! This sensory ability is lost with the use of a needle gun.

ENHANCING THE EFFECTIVENESS OF ACUPUNCTURE

New practitioners may use the same group of points as a senior practitioner yet notice that they are not getting the same results. The following tips look like very basic technique. But these details are important to emphasise. When we understand the rationale behind the technique, we can pay attention to the finer points of needling, which will greatly improve the effectiveness of treatment.

Tonifying first

Reducing tends to be faster and easier than tonification, which usually takes longer to produce an effect. It's like working on a garden; sweeping out the debris shows faster results than planting the landscape. To ensure the best response to treatment, insert tonifying needles first and reducing needles second.

Varying the number of needles

A patient's response will commonly reach a plateau at some point. This is because people's bodies tend to get used to any prescription that has been used for a long series of treatments. So it is a good idea to vary the number and location of points used from time to time, to ensure the patient's continued response to treatment. If you have been using a large number of needles, try some treatments with only a few. Patients who have been seeing a practitioner at regular intervals over a long period of time may need more stimulation, and therefore more needles, than the average person in order to feel a treatment effect.

Optimum length of needle retention

As you know, 15 to 30 minutes is usually long enough to leave the needles in place, except for special circumstances in which the ideal retention time may be shorter or longer. For people with pain from cancer, or a severe migraine, it is not uncommon for an acupuncture session to last as long as 2 hours.

However, for the average patient, a longer treatment is not a better treatment. Researchers have found that after a needle is in for longer than about 45 minutes, the brain will begin to produce an antimorphine-like substance, which will actually reverse the relaxing and therapeutic effects of the treatment. This groundbreaking work was done by Dr Han Jisheng (1998), the famous academician from the Beijing University Neuroscience Research Institute, who led a group of professors and doctors in a major study of the effects of acupuncture on brain chemistry.

Giving attention to needle stimulation

Yes, this is basic technique. However, when newer practitioners or health professionals in fields other than TCM wonder why they are not achieving the expected results with acupuncture, it is frequently because they seem to think the needle works all by itself. The practitioner must stimulate the needles sufficiently to keep the de qi alive. The actions of lifting, thrusting, rotating, stroking, etc. need not be overly strong or aggressive, but should be constantly attended to.

Staying on the line of the meridian

In classical acupuncture, experienced practitioners say they would rather miss the point than miss the line of the meridian. That means that their aim with the needle can be slightly off, as long as it is placed along the meridian. But if the needle hits a point on either side, even if it is only fractionally out of line, this is not acceptable and will not produce the desired treatment effect. The energy flow along the meridian is more important than any individual point. It is like catching the bus – if you don't get it at one stop you can run to the next, but if you're waiting a block off the bus route, you won't get anywhere! Just one of many examples of this is LU-3. The textbook says this point is on the arm, three inches below the end of the axillary fold, on the radial side of the biceps brachii muscle. If a patient has big biceps, the textbook location would place the point too far off the meridian. The point should be aligned with the meridian. Acupuncturists need to train themselves to keep the meridian in their mind's eye at all times while choosing points.

Locating points accurately and efficiently

A large part of your self-education process for the first couple of years of practice is to become absolutely familiar with all the anatomical landmarks that lead to the quickest and most efficient point location. It is much quicker to use your own hands to estimate distance from these reference points than to fiddle about with a measuring tape, especially since any given patient's body is likely to vary from the specific measurements commonly given in English language textbooks. The development of mature technique involves learning the relief map that is made up of the bony processes of the body, and training your eyes to account for variations in anatomy.

Common point location shortcuts include using interlocking hands to find LU-7, under the index finger, or using one hand to cup the patient's knee to locate SP-10 under the tip of your thumb. Another example is GB-34; locate the head of the fibula, with your finger draw a horizontal line underneath and a vertical line medially, and the point will be within the intersection (Fig. 9.9).

About empirical points

One way to produce results quickly is to use powerful empirical points that are known to be effective for particular disorders. Practitioners pick these up by experience or consultation with skilled acupuncturists, but oddly enough these points are rarely given in texts. For example, during any regular treatment, 5–10% per cent of patients will get a scratchy throat or a cough, from all the energy starting to move around in the body. To relieve this, you can use your thumbnail to press on LU-10 for a minute on each side.

Figure 9.9 Using the bony process of the knee as a landmark to locate GB-34.

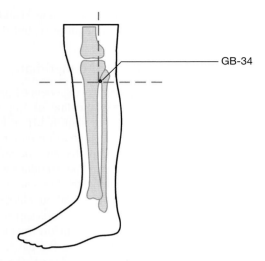

GB-34

Here is a basic set of empirical points. It is not a definitive list; as you do you own research and gain clinical experience you will be able to add your own particular set of tools to this kit to pull out as needed.

Empirical points

- LU-6 – allergic asthma
- LU-11 – sore throat
- LI-18 – hiccups
- ST-7 – acne
- ST-9 – high blood pressure
- ST-34 – weight loss
- ST-45 – dreams that disturb sleep
- HT-5 – excessive sleepiness
- BL-32 – menstrual cramps
- BL-40 – acute lower back injury
- BL-62 – diarrhoea
- LI-3 – frequent urination
- PC-6 – lowering cholesterol and triglycerides
- PC-7 – pain at bottom of heel, including spurs
- TB-17 – migraine
- GB-20 – insomnia
- GB-39 – stiff neck
- GB-40 – pain from shingles
- LIV-2 – anger
- Du-26 – central back pain caused by acute injury
- Ren-9 – water retention
- Ex. Er Bai – haemorrhoids

If you had a traditional Chinese acupuncture teacher, you will have heard the Four Basic Points poem in your first week of training. It is the equivalent of the ABC for acupuncturists, and it is a good start to thinking about empirical points:

The Four Basic Points poem
● Abdomen and stomach, Zu San Li (ST-36) locating
● Waist and back, Wei Zhong (BL-40) begging
● Head and neck, Lie Que (LU-7) seeking
● Face and mouth, He Gu (LI-4) doing

TCM PATTERNS AND WESTERN DIAGNOSIS: MAKING THE LINK

As you know, in TCM there is more than one road to the destination of a diagnosis. When treating a patient, the practitioner looks first at the patient's condition and then progresses to the most appropriate method of diagnosis. In practice, it is important to be familiar with the TCM equivalent for most disorders as described in conventional Western medicine. Most patients who see an acupuncturist arrive with a list of symptoms or a medical diagnosis rather than a TCM pattern. Expect to collect this information gradually, either in your mind or in charts in your treatment room. After several years, you will know most TCM patterns for each main Western disease.

Table 9.1 contains suggestions, drawn from clinical experience and research, for how to begin interpreting Western medical symptoms and diagnoses into Chinese patterns. This is not a definitive list; various practitioners have different views in this area, and you will probably find some new patterns, as human nature is changeable and complicated. An experienced TCM practitioner will be able to incorporate information from a Western diagnosis, with the other conditions observed in the body, as clues to establish the correct TCM pattern for any disease.

Table 9.1 TCM patterns and Western medical diagnoses	
Symptoms/diagnosis	**TCM patterns**
Common cold	Wind-Cold
	Wind-Heat
	Qi deficiency
Headache	Wind-Cold
	Wind-Heat

continued overpage

continued

	Wind–Damp Upsurge of Liver-Fire Liver yang rising Qi deficiency Blood deficiency Kidney deficiency Phlegm obstruction Blood stagnation
Pneumonia	Heat in Lung Phlegm in Lung Dryness injury yin
Diabetes type 2	Heat and Dryness in Lung and injury to Body Fluids Heat in Stomach Spleen and Stomach qi deficiency Kidney yin deficiency Qi and yin deficiency Blood stasis
Overweight	Liver qi stagnation Phlegm-Damp obstruction and Spleen deficiency Stomach Heat obstruction Spleen and Kidney yang deficiency
High cholesterol	Phlegm turbidity blockage Blood stasis Phlegm turbidity blockage with blood stasis Stomach-Heat obstruction Spleen qi deficiency Liver and Kidney yin deficiency Spleen and Kidney yang deficiency
Multiple sclerosis	Phlegm-Damp obstruction Qi and blood stasis Liver and Kidney yin deficiency Kidney yang deficiency
Lupus	Heat and toxic obstruction Yin and blood deficiency Intense Heat toxicity attacking Heart Heat injuring Liver meridian and/or Liver-Wind stirring internally Kidney yin deficiency and blood Heat obstruction Spleen and Kidney yang deficiency

Rheumatoid arthritis	Wind–Cold–Damp impediment (bi) Wind–Heat–Damp impediment (bi) Phlegm obstructing the meridians, and blood stasis Liver and Kidney deficiency (yang and yin)

Asthma	Acute stage
	—Cold type
	—Heat type
	Remission stage
	—Lung and Spleen qi deficiency (root deficiency with
	    branch fullness)
	—Lung and Kidney qi and yin deficiency (root
	    deficiency with branch fullness)

Chronic ulcerative colitis	Downpour of Damp-Heat Hyperactive Liver depressing Spleen, and Spleen deficiency Qi stagnation and blood stasis Spleen and Kidney yang deficiency Yin and blood deficiency
Chronic diarrhoea	Spleen and Stomach qi deficiency Kidney yang deficiency Emotional depression by Liver qi stagnation
Constipation	Dryness-Heat Qi stagnation Blood deficiency and Dryness Qi deficiency Congealing Cold
Irritable bowel syndrome	Phlegm stasis and Liver depression Qi stagnation and Liver depression Heat and Dryness obstruction and Liver depression Damp obstruction and Liver depression
Chronic hepatitis (may include B, C or D)	Heat-Damp obstruction Cold-Damp obstruction Liver yin and Spleen qi deficiency Qi stagnation and blood stasis
Bladder infection	Damp-Heat Blood Heat causing blood in urine

continued overpage

continued

	Downpour of Damp-turbidity
	Kidney and Spleen deficiency
Anaemia	Liver and Heart blood deficiency
	Spleen qi deficiency
	Kidney yang deficiency
High blood pressure	Upsurge of Liver-Fire
	Liver yang rising (yin deficiency with yang hyperactivity)
Hypothyroidism	Spleen and Kidney yang deficiency
	Heart and Kidney yang deficiency
	Hyperactive Liver depressing Spleen
Ménière's disease	Phlegm-turbidity obstructing Spleen
	Spleen qi deficiency
	Liver yang rising
	Kidney yin deficiency
Sciatica	Wind-Cold-Damp impediment (bi)
	Downpour of Damp-Heat
	Qi stagnation and blood stasis
Restless leg syndrome	Blood deficiency and blood stagnation
	Liver and Kidney yin deficiency
	Qi and blood deficiency
Osteoarthritis	Fixed pain impediment (bi)
	Travelling pain impediment (bi)
	Heat attacking meridian impediment (bi)
Frozen shoulder	Qi stagnation and blood stasis
	Congealing Cold and blood deficiency
Premenstrual syndrome	Liver depression and qi stagnation
	Blood deficiency and Liver hyperactivity
	Spleen and Kidney yang deficiency
Endometriosis	Qi stagnation and blood stasis
	Congealing Cold and blood stagnation
	Congealing Heat and qi stagnation
Menopausal syndrome	Liver and Kidney yin deficiency
	Spleen and Kidney yang deficiency

	Liver depression and qi stagnation
	Disharmony of Heart Fire and Kidney water functions
Infertility	Kidney qi deficiency
	Liver depression and qi stagnation
	Qi stagnation and blood stasis
Vaginal yeast infection	Downpour of Damp-Heat
	Liver and Kidney yin deficiency
Allergic sinusitis	Wind-Cold attack and Lung qi deficiency
	Spleen and Lung qi deficiency
	Heat obstruction in Lung meridians
	Kidney qi deficiency, or with Kidney yin/yang deficiency
Chronic fatigue	Spleen qi deficiency (Middle Burner qi deficiency)
	Kidney and Liver yin deficiency
	Yin and yang deficiency
Fibromyalgia	Qi stagnation and blood stasis (meridian and muscle pain)
	Heart and Kidney not communicating
	Liver depression and Liver qi stagnation

References

Han Jisheng 1998 Acupuncture analgesia: fundamentals of neurochemistry. Hubei Science and Technology Publishing House, Wuhan

The practical use of herbs

10

Some readers may be wondering why there is a chapter on herbs in a book for acupuncturists. The main reason is that herbs are such an important part of TCM treatment that they cannot be left out!

As acupuncture became known to Westerners much earlier than Chinese herbs did, people usually come to a TCM clinic specifically for acupuncture treatment. But all acupuncturists should consider adding herbs to their practice, because they have so many useful roles to play.

Each patient is an individual. If acupuncture does not achieve the effect we are expecting, or results do not appear as quickly as we want, herbs are the next tool we can pull out of our kit of healing modalities. Acupuncture relies on the response of the body to achieve results; often the effect can go only as far as the body allows. But herbs work differently. In many respects, herbs are more specific; they have a stronger effect on particular problems. So acupuncture is better at treating functional illnesses and herbs have a stronger, targeted effect on more advanced pathogenic changes of the body. Using herbs in certain cases is, in fact, necessary for good treatment results.

Reasons to use herbs include:

1.	Herbs are effective. Chinese herbal medicine has a long history, and represents an accumulation of a vast amount of experiential knowledge. In China TCM practice is 80% herbology and only 20% acupuncture. For many diseases, the results of herbal medicine are excellent.

2.	Although we use acupuncture to address a patient's symptoms, we may use herbs to balance their whole constitution. In other words, herbs can augment the effects of acupuncture.

3.   Most herbs are plants; therefore, there are few side-effects (if the cooking method and dosage are correct) and we are able to use them for a long period of time.

4.   Herbs are useful to break through a plateau of improvement, when acupuncture alone is not enough for a difficult case. This is a common situation in clinical practice.

There are, however, some important differences of which you should be aware between Chinese herbology and Western herbal practice. In Western herbology, it is quite often the case that one herb is known to be good for treating a particular condition, for instance echinacea to prevent colds, or St John's Wort for depression and restlessness. But when a practitioner is designing a TCM prescription, it is much more complicated. To treat both the symptoms and root causes of this particular patient's condition, 8 to 12 ingredients must be carefully chosen from the hundreds of possible choices.

If your training included herbology, try to work with herbs right from the beginning of your practice. If you delay for a couple of years, you will forget what you have already learned. If your training has not included herbs, I would caution that it is advisable to study the field thoroughly before attempting to use herbs in treatment. Chinese herbology is an extremely complex system. In some jurisdictions, it is illegal for an acupuncturist to prescribe herbs without having done the requisite training and passed the licensing examination.

HERBAL PATENT MEDICINES AND POWDERS

Some practitioners like to prescribe concentrated herbal powder because it has certain advantages, especially for busy people who have no time to cook decoctions. Concentrated powder is as easy and convenient to use as herbal patent medicines, but retains the benefit of raw herbs, which can be individually prescribed and are therefore more specific and more effective.

Concentrated powder comes in a formula format as well as a single herb format. Prescriptions may be designed by mixing individual ingredients or different formulas together. Concentrated herbal powder may not be as strong as the traditional raw herb combinations, but because it is not as time consuming as the raw herbs, which require as much as 2 hours a day to cook, patients are more likely to use it.

Patent medicines are less strong and less expensive than raw herb teas. They are generally used for convenience and long-term support. There are several situations in which it is preferable to use a patent medicine rather than a raw herb tea:

1.   When a patient has no time or no energy; for example, a business person who is constantly travelling, or an elderly or seriously ill person who cannot cook very much, will find a patent medicine more practical.

2. When a patient who has a long-term chronic condition, he or she can be given a strong raw herb tea to start with, followed by several months of patent medicine. Some conditions in which this strategy can be used are coronary artery disease, diabetes, chronic kidney imbalance, or when a cancer patient is undergoing radiation and chemotherapy.

3. When a patient's acupuncture treatments will be interrupted at length, for instance someone who is out of town for the winter, patent medicines help keep the person's health stable until the next treatment opportunity.

A few years ago, Chinese patent medicines arrived in Western countries along with Asian groceries and produce, and were available only in towns and cities with a Chinatown or TCM practitioners' clinics. Things have changed since then; patent medicines are now sold in health food stores, vitamin shops and by practitioners outside the Chinese community. Patents may also be ordered from herbal stores in the nearest centre with an Asian business district. If ordering a large quantity, it is best to contact an herbal wholesale company in metropolitan centres.

A word of caution here: although practitioners and patients of Asian background have been using certain medicines for generations, and their bodies are habituated to the effects of these herbs, this is not necessarily true of non-Asians, so the strength of the 'textbook' prescriptions for some herbs may have to be reduced to suit the tolerance of Western patients.

In addition, not all of the herbal products available in Chinese stores have been through national health authority approval processes. This situation is changing rapidly as the demand in Western countries for Chinese herbal medicine grows. In the meantime, when prescribing patent medicines it is advisable for the practitioner to be sure that the brands are from reputable companies, have undergone testing for good manufacturing processes, are certified to be the right species and part of the plant, and are guaranteed *not* to contain lead, mercury or Western drugs.

New practitioners often find the choice of thousands of herbal preparations overwhelming. Table 10.1 gives a list of suggestions for effective, easily available patent medications to use as a starting point.

RAW HERB TEAS

Since raw herb teas are the strongest form of these medicines, they are also the most effective. Their major disadvantages are the time and attention needed to prepare decoctions, and their strong smell, which non-Asians often find unpleasant. Many patients would appreciate having their herbs cooked for them for a minimal cost. Providing this service could be shared among a group of practitioners if it is too time consuming for a single person.

Table 10.1 Herbal patent medicines

Suggested herbal patent	Purpose of medicine
1. Chuan Xiong Cha Tiao Wan Ligusticum Tea Adjust Pills	For headache due to invasion of Wind-Cold
2. Yin Qiao Jie Du Pian Lonicera Forsythia Detoxification Tablets	For cold flu
3. Bi Yuan Wan Nasal Sinusitis Pills	For sinusitis
4. Huo Xiang Zheng Qi Wan Agastaches Regulate Qi Pills	For stomach flu
5. Kang Ning Wan (Pill Curing) Healthy Peaceful Pills	For indigestion, especially for children. Early cold, flu
6. Chuan Bei Pi Pa Gao Fritillaria Loquat Syrup	For cough
7. Ren Shen Zai Zao Wan Ginseng Reform Pill	For recovering from a stroke
8. Huang Lian Shang Qing Pian Rhizoma Coptidis Upper Clear Tablets	For heat-related cold/flu, infection and constipation
9. Yu Dai Wan Heal Leukorrhoea Pills	For damp-heat leukorrhoea, and candidiasis
10. Qian Jin Zhi Dai Wan Woman Stop Leukorrhoea Pills	For Spleen/Kidney deficiency with dampness leukorrhoea, yeast infection, and candidiasis
11. Niu Huang Jie Du Pian Cow Gallstone Detoxification Tablets	For clearing fire from the Upper and Middle Burners
12. Liu Shen Wan Six Spirit Pills	For severe sore throat and canker sores (short-term use)
13. Shu Gan Wan Comfort Liver Pills	For Liver qi stagnation
14. Xiang Sha Yang Wei Pian Saussureae Amomi Nourish Stomach Pills	For chronic Stomach pain
15. Xiao Yao Wan Relieve Liver Stagnation Pills	For Liver qi stagnation overacting on the Spleen
16. Fu Fang Dan Shen Pian Compound Salviae Tablets	For blood stagnation in cardio-vascular disease
17. Wu Ji Bai Feng Wan Black Chicken White Phoenix Pills	For endometriosis and dysmenorrhoea and irregular menstruation

18.	Shi Quan Da Bu Wan Ten Complete Big Supplement Pills	For qi and blood deficiency
19.	Bu Zhong Yi Qi Wan Nourish Middle Burner Strengthen Qi Pill	For general qi deficiency (Spleen and Stomach)
20.	Gui Pi Wan Nourish Spleen Pills	For Spleen qi and blood deficiency
21.	Fu Ke Ba Zhen Wan Gynaecology Eight Values Pills	For gynaecological concerns with qi and blood deficiency
22.	Liu Wei Di Huang Wan Six Herb Rehmannia Pills	For Kidney and Liver Yin deficiency with Empty Fire
23.	Jin Gui Shen Qi Wan Golden Box Kidney Qi Pills (Sexoton pills)	For Kidney yang deficiency
24.	Yu Chuan Wan Jade Stone Fountain Pills	For diabetes (Type II) with Kidney Yin deficiency
25.	Suan Zao Ren Tang Pian Ziziphi Decoction Tablets	For insomnia and uneasiness

Once a prescription for a raw herb tea has been chosen, the next question is how the patient acquires the herbs. Some practitioners carry a selection of raw herbs commonly used in their practice and sell these directly to patients, though this gives the practitioner the ethical responsibility to be absolutely sure the recommendation of herbs is based on the needs of the patient and not the practitioners' desire to augment their income. Patients may be wary of a practitioner who appears to be trying to get them to spend more money, so it is good to give them other options to purchase the herbs if you can.

The practitioner can order the prescription from an herbal store inside or outside the local community. Or a prescription can be written out and given to the patient to take to the local herbalist. It is also helpful to give the patient a photocopy of the page in your reference book with the herbs and their dosages and write down how many packages are needed. If a range of dosage is given, circle the smaller dosage for frail, very old adults or very young patients, and the larger dosage for younger or more robust adults. Be careful about amounts if you send your patient to an herbal store in Chinatown, as they often use the old system of measurement (1 qian = 3.125 grams). In Western stores and in mainland China, herbalists use grams.

Patients or caregivers who will be cooking raw herbs themselves need clear and simple instructions, preferably written rather than verbal. A handout with blanks to fill in as appropriate should include these important points:

1.   how many times to cook one package of raw herbs
2.   for each cooking, how much water to use and how many cups of tea will be prepared from this process
3.   the cooking time, which depends on the nature of the raw herb tea prescription and how much heat is used in cooking it
4.   information on how often they should drink this tea.

If a patient needs raw herb tea for an extended period of time, practitioners can either order the prescription in powdered form, or grind the herbs themselves and then teach the patient to cook this powder for 10 minutes, or less, before drinking. Another alternative is to sift the powdered herbs finely and put them into gelatine capsules purchased from health food stores. Check the local regulations, though; patients are generally allowed to make capsules for themselves.

Table 10.2 gives a list of important raw herb tea prescriptions for frequently encountered disorders.

EXTERNAL-USE HERBAL PRODUCTS

In your clinic, you may use some liniments and ointments, and you may wish to give some external-use herbal products to your patients. Table 10.3 gives five commonly used external plasters, liniments and ointments.

FOLLOWING UP WITH HERBAL PRESCRIPTIONS

It is always a good idea to check whether the patient is actually taking the herbs as prescribed. Sometimes patients will not understand the practitioner's directions and take the wrong dose at the wrong times. Some patients are afraid of side-effects or drug interactions and don't want to offend you, so they just don't take them. Many patients also have trouble remembering to take medicines three times a day. Some practitioners show patients a chart of blood levels to demonstrate the importance of maintaining blood levels of herbs.

Although it is true that the initial prescription of herbs is very important, it is equally important to interpret the patient's response to them correctly and to make adjustments to the original prescription. Follow-up treatments require complex judgements. The practitioner can try to answer the following questions:

● Is the patient truly better?
● Is the herbal formula producing the desired balancing effect, or is there only a partial effect?
● Should more time be allowed to pass to see the true effect of these herbs?

Table 10.2 Raw herb teas

Raw herb teas to know	Purpose of raw herb tea
1. Ba Zhen Tang The Eight Precious Ingredients Decoction	For qi and blood deficiency
2. Ba Zheng San Powder of Eight Ingredients to Correct Urinary Disturbances*	For urinary tract infections
3. Bai Tou Weng Tang Decoction of Pulsatilla	For diarrhoea from food poisoning
4. Bu Zhong Yi Qi Tang Decoction for Reinforcing the Middle Warmer and Replenishing the Vital Qi	For general qi deficiency (Spleen and Stomach)
5. Chuan Xiong Cha Tiao San Decoction or Tea with Ligusticum	For headache due to invasion of Wind-Cold
6. Dan Dao Pai Shi Tang Biliary Lithagogue Decoction	For gallstones (calculi in the bile duct)
7. Dao Chi San* Powder to Conduct the Heart Fire Downward	For urinary tract infections
8. Ding Chuan Tang Decoction for Asthma	For Heat-related asthma
9. Du Huo Ji Sheng Tang Decoction of Pubescent Angelica and Loranthus	For chronic rheumatic arthritis
10. Er Chen Tang Decoction of Two Herbs-Citrus Peel and Pinellia	For cough with Damp-Phlegm
11. Ge Xia Zhu Yu Tang Decoction to Remove Blood Stasis Below the Diaphragm	For blood stasis due to injury
12. Gui Pi Tang Decoction to Strengthen the Heart and the Spleen	For Spleen qi and blood deficiency
13. Huai Hua San Powder of Sophora Flowers	For bleeding haemorrhoids
14. Ping Wei San The Stomach Neutralising Powder	For stomach pain due to Dampness
15. Sang Ju Yin Decoction of Mulberry Leaf and Chrysanthemum	For Wind-Heat common cold
16. Shen Ling Bai Zhu San Powder of Ginseng, Poria and White Atractylodes	For chronic diarrhoea

continued

17.	Shu Jing Huo Xue Tang Decoction for Removing Blood Stasis in the Channels	For blood stagnation meridian pain
18.	Tian Ma Gou Teng Yin Decoction of Gastrodia and Uncaria	For headache due to Liver yang rising
19.	Tong Xie Yao Fang Powder of White Atractylodes and White Peony for Diarrhoea with Abdominal Pain	For chronic diarrhoea due to Liver qi stagnation
20.	Wu Ling San Powder of Five Drugs with Poria	For chronic oedema
21.	Xiao Chai Hu Tang Minor Bupleurum Decoction	For long-term cold flu
22.	Xiao Yao San Relieve Liver Stagnation Powder/ The Ease Powder	For Liver qi stagnation overacting on the Spleen
23.	Xin Yi San Powder of Magnolia Flower	For sinusitis
24.	Xing Su San Powder of Apricot Seed and Perilla	For chronic cough and Wind-Cold bronchitis
25.	Yi Guan Jian The Liver Reinforcing Decoction	For Liver and Kidney yin deficiency and qi stagnation
26.	Yin Qiao San Powder of Lonicera Flower and Forsythia	For Wind-Cold common cold
27.	Yu Ping Feng San The Jade Screen Powder	For wei qi deficiency, or constant common colds
28.	Zhen Wu Tang Decoction of Zhen-Wu, the God who Control Water	For Spleen and Kidney yang deficiency, and chronic oedema

*These prescriptions classically include Mu Tong, also known as clematis armandi, aristolochia manshuriensis, akebia stem or caulis. Because in larger doses it can cause kidney failure, it is now banned in some countries. Therefore this ingredient should be removed from the prescriptions given. The prescriptions are still good even without Mu Tong.

The knowledge and sensitivity to judge what is really happening are slowly acquired through experience. At first using a classical formula as found in herbal texts will provide a sound basis for herbal prescriptions in accordance with the diagnosis. Then adjustments in dosage and modifications in choice of herbs can be carefully explored. If too many changes are made at once, it will be difficult

Table 10.3 External plasters, liniments and ointments

Product		Use
1.	Zheng Gu Shui Setting-bone Solution	For injuries and arthritic pain
2.	Bao Xin An Po Sum on Oil	For massage, to warm and to promote circulation
3.	Jing Wan Hong Capital City Many Red Colour	For burns, chronic peeling skin, and bedsores
4.	Fu Fang Tu Jin Pi Ding Complex Pseudoljarix Kaempferi (Goldenlarch) Bark Tincture	For fungal skin infections of the feet and hands

to assess what is most effective. Each individual case is an opportunity to practice the art of making these complex decisions within the principles of TCM.

Interpreting patients' responses is also important for the practitioner's understanding of what is truly happening. Initially, patients may be impressed with the incredible amount of detail and the types of questions asked of them, the tongue examination and the reading of their pulses. Patients hope to be helped and approach the practitioner in different ways. Those who are strongly rational tend to report only definite and dramatic changes. Their caution may mislead the practitioner into thinking that the herbal treatment is not working well. However, the tongue and pulse pictures will give their own evidence of change. Other patients desire to present good news and may inaccurately report the effects of the herbs owing to their optimism. Still other patients focus on details to emphasise their concern with their problems and neglect alleviated symptoms in larger, longer-term ways.

Cultivating acceptance and non-judgement of patients is extremely beneficial for practitioners, whichever healing modality is being used. Indirectly these attitudes elicit the same attitudes in patients. In other words, patients who do not feel pressured to *change* because they feel cared for *as they are* are more likely to relax and allow the healing changes to occur. If patients sense that none of their symptoms are bad or wrong, they will report them more objectively and honestly. Practitioners can encourage patients to take notes over time, especially for those who are liable to forget the pattern of changes. However, detail-oriented patients who tend to lose track of general larger changes may not benefit by taking notes. In general, pay attention to both the 'root' cause and the 'branches' symptoms in alignment with the diagnosis, and re-evaluate your diagnosis if the treatment results are unsatisfactory.

Opening a clinic

11

When you graduate from acupuncture college or finish your training programme and you wish to set up a practice, you need to know whether you are mentally and emotionally ready to focus and commit yourself to it. This is a career that demands devotion for years, for a lifetime. It is better not to dabble in acupuncture. You are dealing with the serious matter of people's health and well-being, and your failure or success with patients affects them and their families. When you want to make this commitment and feel happy to do so, you will find that your work is really a mutual energy flow between you and your patients.

You are more likely to feel ready to open a clinic when you have had enough hours of needling practice, when you have had experience with many different patient conditions and when you can make a correct TCM diagnosis 70–80% of the time. Regulatory bodies in different jurisdictions have their own minimum internship periods.

Remember that the first year of practice is always a growing experience. Expect business to be slow; this is normal. Planning well and doing your research will get your practice off to a good start. The following section touches on the basic business issues a TCM practitioner needs to consider; more in-depth information is available in many excellent books and community education classes. Governments often have programmes to assist new businesses as well.

BEGINNING WELL – LEGALITIES, LOCATION AND LOGISTICS

Before starting a clinic, there are many things to think about. The first question to ask yourself is what is your dream practice? What do you want your clinic to be like? People who have a clear and well thought out vision of what they want to achieve are far more likely to be successful than those who just muddle along day to day with no concrete plan.

Imagine what your clinic will be like when it is established, 1 year from now, and 3 or 5 years down the road. Working from home is different from having a clinic in a professional building. A practice in which the acupuncturist does everything including answering the phone and emptying the wastebasket is different from sharing office space with multiple practitioners and a receptionist. The decision on the structure of your practice will influence your choice of location and the size of the clinic space you will need.

Licensing and insurance

An acupuncture clinic in many ways is no different from any other kind of business. It is important, right from the beginning, to figure out what kind of business arrangement suits you best: a sole proprietorship, a partnership or incorporation. There are many issues of taxation and liability involved in this decision. For instance, if someone sued you, would your home and other personal assets be vulnerable, or just your business? Taxation and liability laws vary from country to country. Before you open your door to patients, it is wise to consult a qualified accountant or financial adviser about how to set up your practice and your financial records. A small expenditure at this crucial time can save you money and prevent problems in the future.

Depending on the area in which you live, you may be required to have two licences to practise: one from a regulatory body such as an acupuncture or TCM college, the other from your local or regional government. In many countries, acupuncturists must be licensed by an official registration body, much like a College of Physicians and Surgeons. In order to practise in these jurisdictions, you have to fulfil certain requirements. The regulations set out the minimum number of years of study, length of internship, treatment of a certain number of patients, and completion of some mandatory courses, as well as passing final examinations.

Whereas some jurisdictions now have a well-developed examination, licensing and registration process, others do not. It is the practitioners' responsibility to research the regulations in the area where they wish to practise. Even where there are no government regulatory bodies, it is a good idea to join the nearest professional association, so that patients have some assurance that the practitioner is properly qualified.

Also, municipalities, cities or counties will probably require you to have a business licence. Some will have a category for acupuncturists; in other areas you may be in the category of health consultants or medical services. Local governments will, in addition, have laws governing zoning for businesses, including health care offices. The regulations cover the location of your office (it may or may not be legal for you to practise in your home), as well as signs, hours of operation, parking spaces, etc.

Make sure, before you open your clinic, that you are covered by malpractice insurance, to protect your patients and yourself. Your professional organisation or college can help you find a practitioners' group insurance plan, which will cover you for a more reasonable cost than an individual insurer. Another kind of insurance to look into is general liability coverage for the premises in which you practise. This would cover situations such as someone falling down your stairs. Offices available for rent in medical buildings may already carry such coverage, but it is wise to check. If your clinic is in your home, you will need liability insurance, either as part of your general home-owner coverage, or as extra business insurance.

Choosing a location

Choosing a location for your practice first involves picking the right community, and then deciding where in that community to open your clinic. Take time to research and think about your options. It is better to spend 2 or 3 months deciding on a location than moving here and there, hoping your patients will be willing to follow.

In choosing a geographical area, consider the factors of population size and how many acupuncturists are already practising there. In the far Western part of Canada, for instance, practitioners have observed that a community with a population of 4000–5000 people is the minimum required to support one full-time acupuncturist. If there are 10 000 residents in an area within a reasonable driving distance of the clinic, two good acupuncturists should be able to support themselves. People from outlying areas may come in for treatment, but aren't likely to become regular enough patients to make a difference in the viability of a practice. Of course, the ideal ratio of practitioner to population won't be the same in the south of England or California as it is in the Australian outback, but the basic principle of looking for a situation where demand is higher than supply holds true everywhere.

New graduates tend to stay in crowded towns or cities and therefore may find it difficult to build a practice. Parts of the country where there are few practitioners often hold the most potential for establishing a successful new practice. To find out how many practitioners are in an area, consult the membership listings of a large acupuncture association with hundreds of members, or collect the telephone directory and check the business pages. The city or town hall's business licence department may also be able to help you.

Next, find out who are the existing acupuncturists in the area. What are their specialities? Is one a physiotherapist who occasionally performs acupuncture, or a full-time acupuncture practitioner? Ideally you could go there and meet these practitioners. This way you could find out whether the local population's need for their services is greater than the existing practitioners can supply, whether they plan any major life changes, such as moving out of the area, or whether they are open to sharing the patient load. Perhaps they would rather teach taiji than practise acupuncture! By looking more deeply into each situation, you may uncover a wonderful opportunity to support each other's practice.

Also consider the economic status and main employers of the area, and the average age and racial background of the populace. These factors may influence your choice of location because they will affect the nature of your practice. Are there likely to be many people with industrial injuries, a high level of alcoholism, or many with respiratory problems or who wish to quit smoking? Perhaps you would prefer a community popular with retirees because you are interested in treating people with heart conditions, poststroke syndrome, or prostate problems, or you'd enjoy a family-oriented suburb because you want to focus on women's health concerns. The economic stability of the community is an important factor to consider as well. For example, if most of the local population is employed by one company and that company closes down, this spells radical change for the local economy.

Having an established network of friends and family can be an important drawing factor to an area. If you have lived there previously, you already know the social structure and general concerns of the people. For example, a woman who had pursued a career in business left her home city to study acupuncture and returned 3 years later to open a practice; it was successful because she still had a network of business contacts there.

Try to visit the area you are interested in at least a few times, telephone people, read about the place and get a sense of the population's general attitude towards alternative medicine. Notice how many health food stores there are, what sorts of festivals they celebrate, and whether the library carries any books on acupuncture.

CULTURAL CONTEXT

It is important to recognise and to consider the implications of the culture in which you intend to set up your acupuncture practice. In the United Kingdom, parts of Europe and North America, as well as Australia and New Zealand, Asian populations are significant in certain regions or major urban centres and are otherwise less concentrated throughout these countries. Around the Pacific Rim there are areas that have been settled for generations by people of Asian heritage. Where there is a well-established Asian culture, there will probably be Chinese herbal stores as well as food markets and restaurants. This influences the local culture by exposing people to the possibility of Chinese medicine. Other cultures such as Indian may have strong roots in an area and bring their own health care traditions, such as Ayurvedic medicine, to their local communities.

The advantage of cultural exposure is greater familiarity with the ideas and practices of acupuncture, better access to herbal supplies and a community of people whose upbringing included acupuncture and herbs. Conversely, the advantage of establishing an acupuncture clinic in an area with very little Asian culture is that you become an ambassador of TCM with the opportunity to educate people well right from the start. A man from Ohio who saw me in Victoria whilst visiting relatives told me that there was no acupuncturist within 200 miles of his home. An acupuncturist setting up in this man's town would have to start from scratch in educating the local populace, but the reward would be the opportunity to build a strong, healthy practice with little or no competition.

Whatever geographic area you choose for your clinic, researching the cultural groups present will help you to understand their probable exposure to different health practices and enable you to serve their needs more effectively.

LOCATING YOUR OFFICE

The location of your office can significantly affect the success of your practice. Most important is that your office is reasonably easy to find. Secondly, it should be easily accessible by car or public transportation. Two blocks' walking distance is too much for some elderly and infirm patients. Thirdly, parking must be easily available because the stress of difficult parking will discourage people from coming to see you if there is an easier option.

What is the inside of the office like? Consider the following points:

- Is there a window for air and light to uplift patients' spirits – not to mention those of the practitioner?
- Is there enough room for a properly set up treatment area, storage of supplies, secure storage of patient records?
- Is the clinic accessible to patients with impaired mobility or those in wheelchairs? If it isn't at ground level, there should be an elevator.
- Lastly, but also important, is it a peaceful and quiet location? Patients will not be able to relax during their treatments if they are surrounded by the din of traffic or a factory next door.

Graduates often ask whether it is acceptable to practise at home or from their parents' basement. This depends on municipal zoning regulations, which may designate a neighbourhood as residential only or permitting medical therapy. Check whether you are allowed to put up a sign by the street or one in the window. Think about the peace of your treatment room with respect to house noise (loud music, creaky water pipes, or people walking around heavily). Consider the availability of parking, and make sure your home situation has a convenient and accessible washroom. If you do practise at home, it is best not to mix telephone lines; have a separate telephone number for work.

The benefits of a practice at home are saving money you would otherwise spend on renting an office space, and the convenience of looking after house affairs or arranging for child care more easily. Especially on islands or in rural areas, where people are used to home-based or cottage businesses, a separate or attached treatment room in the family dwelling is fine. However, attitudes are different in cities. Urban residents may believe a home-based practice is less formal or even less professional, and they may be concerned about their privacy with respect to other members of the household.

You, as a practitioner, may choose an office away from home because you value your personal and family privacy. There is the possibility that patients will knock on your house door to see you at any time they wish (in which case a sign indicating 'by appointment only' and indicating office hours is in order). It may be that locking the door of a professional building at the end of the day allows you to leave your work stress behind.

However, a home-based practice is something to consider seriously, especially for the first 6 months to a year. It will decrease your financial pressures and you can relocate to a rented office if you choose when you have already built up clientele.

However, do not choose your office location or move your clinic without careful consideration. With each move you make, you will lose some patients and create stress for those who remain with you. People tend to feel more relaxed and at peace in familiar, stable surroundings. If there are problems with your current location, try to solve them in other ways before you contemplate moving. If relocation is absolutely necessary, try to give your patients sufficient notice and information.

Expanding your clinic

An acupuncture clinic often opens with one person playing multiple roles. You are the doctor, receptionist and office manager. You not only have to be a good therapist, but summon the time and energy for filing, organising, marketing and even tidying up.

As the practice grows, it is good to be prepared to expand the enterprise by handing over some of the roles. Usually this means hiring a receptionist. This allows you to be free from booking appointments, billing and receiving, answering phones, advertising, ordering supplies, etc., and gives you more time to focus on your knowledge, skills and business growth. However, businesses often fail when they expand too quickly. Staff salaries and benefits are a significant expense so be sure that your practice can support the extra expenditure first.

Expansion can also mean sharing the office with other health care practitioners, such as a massage therapist, herbalist, chiropractor or naturopath. These may be an excellent complement to your services and a great convenience to your clients when they need some other form of treatment. At the same time, it can help to keep the clinic's overhead costs down, especially if several practitioners can share a receptionist or office manager.

CREATING A UNIQUE STYLE AND ENVIRONMENT

Naming your clinic

The name of your clinic is largely a matter of personal preference, but should reflect the way you wish to portray yourself and the services you offer to your prospective client base. What is your mission statement? What are you most excited about offering to your patients? What is it that makes you different from other acupuncturists?

You may think it is difficult to create something very much different from what other practitioners offer, simply because you are doing pretty much the same work. But contemplating your own strengths, cultural background, education, special knowledge or skills, even your personality and interests, will help you create a unique professional image. This image tells people what is special about you and your practice.

When you begin, it may be best not have a name for your clinic other than a descriptor like 'Acupuncture and herbal clinic' so that you leave yourself room to change and to expand. The most appropriate name also depends on location. For example, in a professional building you may want simply to use your name and your credentials (Registered or Licensed Acupuncturist, Diploma of TCM, or Dr TCM, depending on the regulations in your area). A name that relates to your location is also short, informative and easy to remember.

You may want to choose a less prosaic name for your clinic when you focus on a specific area of practice. For example, 'Kuan Yin Acupuncture and Herbal Clinic', named for a kind-hearted female Buddha, is appropriate for a clinic focusing on women's health concerns.

If you are establishing a retreat centre in a place of natural beauty, where meditation, qigong, taiji, acupressure, tui na, acupuncture, or some combination of therapies will be offered, a well-chosen descriptive name is essential in creating an image that will attract clients. Every temple in China, Japan and Korea has a name indicating a place of retreat, a spiritual home or a restful natural environment.

Be careful to avoid misunderstanding, or setting up incorrect expectations in people's minds about your treatments based on the name you give your clinic. For example, someone may think a spirit-related name means that you treat only psychological and emotional disorders. An overly long or fancy name, or one that requires translation or background knowledge, will not stick in people's minds.

Once you've settled on a few possibilities, do a name search at your local or regional business registry to see whether anyone else in the area is already using them. Be aware that if you are not incorporated, your use of a business name may not be protected, even if you have been using it for years.

Creating an individual practice style

Style is far easier to sense than it is to explain, but it is something that every practitioner needs to think about and develop. The institution you have attended will have trained you in a particular style or 'school' of acupuncture. But style is more than that.

You could say that style is everything that makes your practice *your* practice. You could also say that style is your way of 'being' in your practice. Through your style, you express your vision, your intention and your purpose in doing this work. A caution for new practitioners who have not yet fully developed their own style is the tendency to adopt, temporarily, whichever one they've most recently encountered in workshops or seminars. This can be disconcerting to patients who will never know what to expect at the next visit.

For this reason, a major element of style is having a consistent and unique approach that draws patients to you. It is your manner of greeting and relating with your patient. It is your way of diagnosing and your technique. It is the atmosphere you create in your treatment room and with your personality. It is your degree of formality and your level of detail or generality. Thus, some of the qualities that constitute style are simply who you are, whereas other qualities are nurtured and formed, such as the atmosphere you create. Patients come to know your ways, and their trust grows. They are usually reluctant to change practitioners because they are familiar with your style.

The style of practice with which you feel comfortable is of course influenced by your own family, cultural and educational background. Another factor is your patients' general expectations and interests – what makes *them* feel comfortable. You need both to respect your patients and to find a way to meet them in their familiar world.

Style is also affected by the geographical area of your practice. You need to suit and to balance, or counteract the imbalances of, the area. For example, your office in a busy city could be a quiet sanctuary, with pictures of nature on the walls, and yet you may wear more formal clothing to suit your patients who have a business or professional background.

The presence of acupuncture colleges teaching certain styles of acupuncture will influence the expectations of people living in the surrounding community. For example, the renowned Professor J. R. Worsley combined Chinese and Japanese elements and his own method to develop a Five Elements style widely used in treatment of emotional and psychological issues; he founded the College of Traditional Chinese Acupuncture in the UK and the Traditional Acupuncture Institute in the US. Schools in many other countries offer courses in Five Elements style along with classic TCM. Other centres specialise in Japanese or Korean styles of acupuncture.

Since the colleges have student clinics, local people may directly experience treatments and others will hear about treatments from friends. Depending on their evaluation of the treatments, they may have a favourable or unfavourable opinion of that style of acupuncture, which may then spill over to the way they view your practice. Providing the same style of acupuncture as a local student clinic may at first be difficult for your business since clients would receive a supervised treatment for less cost at the student clinic. However, as your experience grows there will be clients who prefer to visit your professional and peaceful clinic despite the greater cost.

For the first 1½ to 2 years, you will be very consciously forming your own approach and, with further training, be influenced by schools of acupuncture other than the one you were exposed to first. Many acupuncturists find that it works best to build on their roots in a consistent manner rather than becoming too scattered or eclectic, a 'Jack of all trades' who does not know one way deeply.

Clearly communicating to patients which style you practise will help them to know what to expect or at least to be open to what you have to offer. It will also help you focus your marketing; this discussion continues in the next chapter.

Creating your clinical environment

Clinical environments can be quite varied, depending on where you practise, the needs and expectations of the patients you want to attract, and your own style (Fig. 11.1). Some practitioners like to maintain a strictly professional, medical environment. Others like to create a soothing, Asian-inspired spa-like setting complete with flute music, incense, plants and a water fountain.

Beautiful artwork or photos can help patients to feel relaxed. Good diagrams of acupuncture points and meridians are useful in explaining concepts

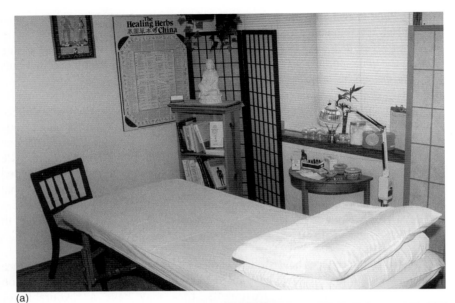

(a)

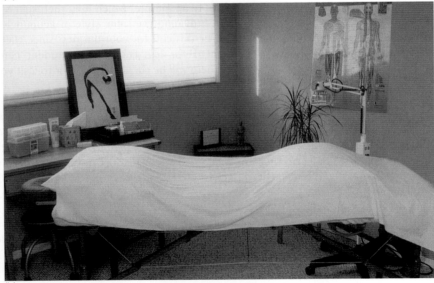

(b)

Figure 11.1a and b Typical clinic settings.

to patients, or in helping patients describe their symptoms to you, for example by showing you their radiation of pain. Likewise, you could use an acupuncture doll.

Appropriate lighting is critical. Avoid overhead lighting; use lamps, halogen lights or, best of all, natural light through windows whenever possible. Always adjust window blinds to suit patients' needs and emotional and spiritual comfort.

Sound is best kept to a minimum. Music played very quietly may be all right when treating muscular disorders or sleep disorders, but may not be appropriate in many cases. Soft music in a soundproof waiting room is generally acceptable, unlike a radio news broadcast, which is unlikely to be conducive to patients' peace of mind and relaxation.

Your choice of wording and delivery is very important in creating a relaxed atmosphere. Slowing down and being calm is part of your treatment. From you, patients could learn how to stop rushing. Watch the feeling of time pressure in yourself, and take care not to project this outward in the presence of your patient. If patients feel rushed, they could fall down or their blood pressure might increase, and they will certainly enjoy their treatment less than if they feel relaxed about time.

Adjust your planned schedule in your mind in order to let go of worry and time pressure. If someone arrives late, nothing can change that. It is best to let go of irritation and do the best job you can. Concentrate your efforts in the shorter period of time you have by using acupressure and tui na, in addition to acupuncture, or you could ask fewer questions and continue with a good acupuncture treatment. Remember that your gentle voice and kind attitude may be the most important part of the treatment for someone.

Naturally, a clean and neat environment is important to build safety and trust with your patients. That includes your person as well as the treatment room. Unless you are practising in an unusually casual environment, your patients will feel more confident if your dress is appropriate, which is generally at the same level of formality or informality as your clients. Some practitioners like to wear a lab coat; others prefer to look less medical. You must always be clean, have clean hair and fingernails and be well-groomed. Keep a toothbrush and other grooming accessories at the office for touch-ups during the day.

SELF-CARE FOR THE PRACTITIONER

A healthy clinical environment requires a practitioner who is healthy in body, mind and spirit. Our stamina and relaxation will be supported by taking the following steps to take care of ourselves. It is much like the common sense advice we give our patients, but as we know it takes some work and commitment to make these things a habit.

Schedule your treatment days wisely. This means taking a short break after seeing three or four patients, rather than pushing through half a dozen before stopping. In your breaks, have a snack, a drink of water or cup of tea. Don't just close your door and read a magazine – go outside if at all possible and take a walk. Even 10 minutes of moving around and getting some air will clear the mind.

Take vacations!

Be sure to empty your bladder from time to time. When we get busy, our brain ignores signals from the bladder and we retain urine for too long. This can cause bladder infections or even, in the long term, kidney damage.

Try not to spend hours on the computer at the end of the work day. After hours of treating patients, your back, arms, legs and brain will be tired and sitting at the computer will add more brain and eye strain. Although it is important to write up your patient notes, try to schedule your other office paperwork for a half-day during the week or at the weekend.

Walking, yoga, taiji or qigong are excellent ways to move your body and to clean out the stress and other unhealthy energy you have absorbed from your work. Cultivating a hobby, such as art, music, dancing, athletic activity, etc. is another good way to achieve a healthy balance.

TCM practitioners shouldn't have to be told this, but I know many who do not take the time during the day to nourish themselves. It is imperative to eat regularly, and have a well-balanced diet – not just grab an apple for lunch or wolf down a chocolate bar when energy is flagging. It is also imperative to stay hydrated. No matter how busy we are, we must schedule mealtimes as well as patients, and plan to have healthy meals and snacks on hand. Our ability to think clearly and do effective treatments suffers, especially at the end of the day, if blood sugar is low.

We are healers, but sometimes we need help to heal ourselves. Having other practitioners to 'debrief' with about difficult cases, or other supportive people to talk to about our personal struggles is balm to the spirit, and helps us maintain perspective. It is particularly important to have ways to handle our own grief when a patient dies.

EQUIPMENT AND SUPPLIES FOR THE ACUPUNCTURE CLINIC
Needles

Based on average daily use, below are some general guidelines for stocking supplies of needles, starting from the type of which you'll need the largest quantity and working down. The gauge numbers indicate the thickness of the needle: the bigger the gauge number, the *thinner* the diameter of the needle. In normal clinical use, the thinnest needle we use is gauge 38, which is 0.18 mm in diameter:

- *1 cun (25 mm):* mostly, we use gauge 36 (0.20 mm diameter) and gauge 34 (0.22 mm diameter)
- *2 cun (50 mm):* mostly, we use gauge 34 (0.22 mm diameter) and gauge 32 (0.25 mm diameter); the thinner gauge 34 needles are used in finer-skinned patients
- *0.5 cun (13 mm):* mostly we use gauge 36 (0.20 mm diameter) and gauge 38 (0.18 mm diameter); these needles are best for most points on children, and for some sensitive points on adults

- *3 cun (75 mm):* mostly we use gauge 32 (0.25 mm diameter) and gauge 30 (0.30 mm diameter); these are used for points where muscle and tissue are very thick, such as the hip. The 30 gauge are also used for points where muscle and tissue are thick, and in addition if the patient is very large and muscular.

The treatment table

A good treatment table has a firm, yet comfortable surface, with very stable legs to support it. You will also need to acquire an adjustable head/face rest, as well as removable extensions for the patients' arms, so there is enough room for them to be in a comfortable position. You may also want to have a treatment table that is light and easy to fold down and transport, for occasions when you do workshops or treat people in locations other than your clinic. Check companies that produce massage tables and look at different models before buying or building your table.

Other necessary supplies

These are some suggestions. You will want to modify this list according to your personal situation.

- 70–75 % alcohol for cleaning skin around the acupoints
- 95–99% alcohol for cupping
- Hibitain or a similar cleanser for patients who are allergic to alcohol
- 2–5% iodine, which is very important to have on hand in case you accidentally puncture yourself with a used needle; you never know whether the patient might have hepatitis or HIV, and alcohol and a bandage are not as effective as iodine, so make sure you have this
- Glass cups for cupping: you will need four large, four medium, and four small ones
- Two forceps – one for clean material, one for used; curved forceps are the easiest to use – you'll have to specify this when ordering
- Container for used needles; The proper 'sharps' container should be purchased from a medical supply store, as other kinds of containers may be too easily punctured
- Alcohol dispenser
- Ear beads
- Electrical stimulator
- Moxa sticks, loose moxa, and a glass jar with sand in which to extinguish burning sticks, and in which to fix the incense sticks that you use to light the loose leaves
- Small dish for collecting needles as you are removing them from the patient
- Blood pressure cuff with stethoscope
- Adhesive bandages/sticking plasters

- Footstool, to help patients get on to the table
- General office supplies: receipt book, brochure holders, answering machine, etc.
- Therapeutic lamp: there are many different kinds these days, including infrared, TDP heat, and oscillating frequency lamps (I like the TDP heat lamp because it has both a therapeutic wave effect as well as warmth – see under 'Safety with other techniques', in Section One)
- Massage tincture or oil: some good ones are Zhen Gu Shui (setting-bone solution), or Bao Xin An (Po Sum On Oil) for massage; some practitioners prefer Western herbal massage oils, flower essential oils, etc.
- Diagrams or acupuncture models, and herb posters: these can help you explain your treatment choices to patients; you may also want to put up a notice requesting patients not to wear scents such as perfume or aftershave, as some of your other patients are likely to have allergies to these
- Treatment table linens are a big issue: patients often dislike the disposable paper used by physicians to line their tables, which is endurable for the length of a brief examination but cold and uncomfortable while lying there for a 40 minute treatment; cotton pillow cases and sheets are much more pleasant. It is a good idea to use a small cover on top of the pillowcase and another on the table, which can quickly and easily be changed, especially after treating people who perspire. A couple of light blankets are good to have for when a patient is feeling chilly.

CLINIC REGULATIONS

Below are some suggested regulations for an acupuncture school or a clinic in which an intern or apprentice is working. Having a set of agreed-upon regulations on the wall is also useful in a clinic that is shared with other practitioners. Confusion about the proper disposal of used needles, for example, can lead to injuries and infection.

Clinic regulations

—Clothing and personal grooming should be clean, neat and professional.
—Respect the patients' privacy. Do not discuss their problems in public or with anyone else, unless you are consulting professionally with another practitioner. Uncover only those parts of the patient's body that you must in order to do the treatment.
—Wash your hands before *and* after treating each patient.
—Have separate and clearly labelled areas for clean and contaminated supplies.
—After a treatment is complete, collect all used needles and place immediately and carefully into the designated disposal container.

—Check the floor, the table, the sheets and pillows for lost needles to ensure no one is punctured by accident.

—Always put discarded needles into the sharps container, never into the regular waste basket, and make sure an empty needle package is in fact empty before discarding it into the waste receptacle.

—Turn all dials to zero, turn off and disconnect all electrical devices – lamps, electrical stimulator, etc. – at the end of each treatment.

Basic business management for the acupuncturist

12

PROFESSIONAL AND COMMUNITY NETWORKING

You are opening your clinic in your chosen community, and now you have to let people know about yourself and your practice. Building and nurturing a professional network helps you feel less alone in your practice and more like part of a team. It also enables you to stay up to date with changes in practice, innovations in medicine and health issues in your area. Even if you practise in an outlying community, you still need to nurture this network; in fact it is probably even more important to seek out connections when you are the only acupuncturist for miles.

Registration bodies and professional associations

Colleges of acupuncture and other regulatory bodies exist to protect the public. Your regulatory body will also keep you abreast of developments in the field and any changes in legislation that affect practitioners.

However, it is to your benefit to join also the nearest acupuncture association, which exists to promote the profession, represent members in local, national and international settings, and lobby governments for changes to legislation. Many of these organisations also offer professional development seminars and provide opportunities to form networks with your peers.

Experienced acupuncturists

Networking with other practitioners is crucial to your practice. Once a connection has been established, you may contact them for consultation about difficult cases, to exchange ideas when several treatment options are available, or to refer a patient you have seen because you are unable to treat a particularly serious condition owing to a lack of experience or expertise. You may also recommend people who will be in the experienced practitioner's area to see them. This often occurs with friends and relatives of your patients. Once you make an initial contact with a practitioner, all future dealings proceed more smoothly.

Classmates

After you graduate, keep in touch with your classmates, notifying each other of your changing locations and sharing information. This network can be a strong support. Perhaps you could all write a yearly newsletter, and share this task among yourselves. Two people may even work together in a clinic in a newly developed area. If classmates travel to another country or learn a new technique somewhere, they could inform everyone about their experience.

Medical doctors

Many physicians are becoming more open to complementary health care, especially when qualified practitioners take the time to introduce themselves and tell them a bit about acupuncture. Some doctors may need to know that you are not trying to encourage people to shun Western medicine in favour of TCM. Maintaining a good relationship with your patients' physicians is very valuable in allowing you access to information such as lab results that would give you a broader understanding of the symptoms or disease in question, which ultimately helps you treat your patients more effectively.

When a physician refers a patient to you, and after treating this person for a while you are seeing changes in the condition, this is a good time to get in touch with the doctor and offer an update about what treatments you have done and what the effects have been. It might even be appropriate to request that the doctor reassess the patient's condition and progress and let you know the results. This feedback helps you decide whether to continue with the current treatment plan or to make some modifications. Also, medical doctors generally become more willing to refer people as patients share with them their experiences and the improvements in their health.

In more serious cases, where the patient's condition requires a combined approach between Western and TCM practitioners, it helps to send the physician a letter that outlines the patient's symptoms and progress, and introduces acupuncture with a brief description of how it will help the patient. It is best to avoid using too much TCM terminology or lengthy explanations of the principles of Chinese medicine, which may create confusion in the doctor's mind. Over time, the doctor will see which patients are likely to benefit from acupuncture, and a complementary medical relationship develops. Eventually the physician may want to learn more about TCM.

Send a thank-you note to the doctor, or any other practitioner, who refers a patient to you. And remember to be pleasant and polite to the receptionist, who is the 'gatekeeper' for the doctor. Receptionists who are familiar with you and your practice often quietly recommend you to other people and may even remind the doctor about acupuncture.

Other members of the health care community

One aspect of establishing an acupuncture practice is establishing roots, finding and meeting the people in the community who offer complementary services. These may be other practitioners such as naturopaths, body workers, physiotherapists, chiropractors, counsellors and mental health workers, midwives and menopause educators. Other good contacts are health food and nutritional supplement suppliers, Chinese herbal suppliers, qigong and taiji teachers, and leaders of support groups. Introducing yourself and your services, and learning about what they offer, even offering them a gift certificate for an acupuncture treatment, are all possible ways to build a network of supportive people who know and trust each other's work and therefore feel comfortable referring appropriate patients. Networking requires patience and a long-term view of being part of a community. Remember that people get busy and may forget about you, so it helps to send them a card for Christmas or Chinese New Year, or email them health newsletters or even interesting articles or research studies.

Associations for various diseases

Associations for fibromyalgia, arthritis, cancer, heart disease and stroke, diabetes and other conditions often like to suggest different complementary therapies as options for their members. They may ask you if you would like to be on a list of recommended practitioners, and they generally renew this list every year. This is a helpful way of advertising your clinic.

You could also research one of these conditions and approach the associations, introducing to them the perspective of TCM regarding their condition. Perhaps they will arrange for you to give a seminar for their members and their families.

The community

Schools, community and local activity centres are all great places to network. Whatever you enjoy doing may provide an opportunity to share information about acupuncture. For instance, a practitioner who is interested in ancient Chinese philosophy may practise calligraphy as a hobby. Others in the class may be curious about the practitioner's profession. If at some point later they're looking for an acupuncturist, this connection is likely to come to mind.

If you join an amateur soccer club, your fellow players may well be interested in acupuncture's effectiveness in pain relief for sports injuries! In essence, you are creating a need for your services that these people may never have realised before.

You can also make excellent contacts by joining organisations such as the YMCA/YWCA, Chamber of Commerce, or service clubs like Rotary International. Remember, when networking, that many people no longer appreciate the 'hard sell'. Approach networking with the attitude that you are there to help others connect with whatever resources they need, whether or not that includes an acupuncturist at the moment. You will find that this opens many unexpected doors that will be of benefit to you in the long run. Always carry business cards and be prepared to hand out many of them.

Health is always a pertinent topic in the media, which can be a useful networking tool. You might want to send the local newspaper, radio or TV station a one-page introduction of yourself and your new clinic, expressing a willingness to be telephoned for information if they are ever doing a story on alternative medicine. Also, you can watch their listings and ads for local health-related forums and events in which you could participate.

FOCUSED MARKETING

If you decide to place an advertisement to announce the opening of your new clinic, keep in mind the circulation of the publication. People who live a great distance away are not likely to drive all the way to your clinic unless you are the only practitioner for 200 miles. The local papers may have less prestige but they will reach the people who are most likely to become patients, and for a lower cost.

Focused marketing is more effective, and is a more efficient expenditure of time, effort and money, than trying to sell your services to everyone. This means spending some time to figure out who your ideal patients are and then to market yourself more specifically to them.

The first step is to define what you offer that is unique. Perhaps you have developed a specialty like sports medicine, women's health issues, caring for children or treating skin diseases. Perhaps you are most interested in serving the elderly or in practising in a retreat-like setting. When you know what sets you apart and what you truly want to do, you can better direct your energy to marketing that.

Next, imagine your ideal patient complete with conditions and problems. This will probably be linked with the first step; for example, if you desire to work primarily with the elderly, then your ideal patient may be 70 years old, full of life stories and wisdom, and suffering with Heart and Kidney qi deficiency. The more specific you are about whom you would ideally like to treat, the more clear and effective you will be in advertising and presenting yourself to the public.

When communicating what you offer, whether this is in personal conversation with patients or prospective patients, or in your promotional materials, think in terms of benefits rather than features. For instance, in treating people with back pain, a 'feature' might be that you use special Japanese needles, but patients won't know what that means unless you tell them how this feature is of benefit to them.

The third step is to determine how to reach these people with these conditions. Think about the places this type of patient would go, their habits and their interests. Research the stores, companies and organisations where you think this type of person would spend their time. In this manner you are already beginning to market yourself with your target group of people.

PROMOTIONAL MATERIALS

Self-promotion is often a difficult issue for people in the helping professions. On the one hand, we have to make potential patients aware of our services if our clinic is going to thrive. But we also have an ethical responsibility to represent ourselves in a manner befitting health professionals. Practitioners whose promotional materials make outrageous claims about acupuncture or their own ability to 'cure' people may attract many patients initially, but the patients' inevitable disillusionment can damage not only the practitioner's reputation but the credibility of the profession as a whole.

Always find out how patients found out about you. Did they look under the acupuncturist listing in the yellow pages? Did an acquaintance give them your card? Did they see your brochure at the health food store? This helps you determine your advertising strategy and budget.

Business cards

These days everybody knows about the need for a well-designed business card. Along with your name and contact information, you may want to include your clinic logo. A logo helps you create a recognisable identity for your clinic. Graphics often leave people with a stronger and longer-lasting impression than text. A logo can also be used on your brochure, handouts, appointment cards and on signs outside your office, if appropriate.

Include your qualifications and the name of the regulatory body that has approved them; patients sometimes phone there to check you out. This reassures patients that you have undergone sufficient training and practice to be properly qualified.

Designing an effective brochure

In Chinese it is said, 'a brochure is your clothing'. Therefore, it needs to reflect your knowledge and approach. The style of the words should match the style of your practice. Your purpose is to provide enough information about TCM to help patients get the most benefit from treatment, and enough information about yourself and your way of practising to reassure people that you are offering a safe, professional and effective service.

The general guideline for printed material is to keep it simple and clear, not too fancy and with not too much information. The print size needs to be large enough so that people can read it without digging out their reading glasses (a point that young people often forget!). Too much text in too small a font can feel overwhelming. Also, people are initially more interested in you and what you can do for their health than in the field of acupuncture. After all, they are coming to see you, and if they wished to study Chinese medicine they could borrow good books from most libraries. Here are some suggestions for information that is commonly included in acupuncturists' brochures:

- *Who are you?* What is your professional designation, as in Registered Acupuncturist, Registered TCM Practitioner or Doctor, or whatever qualifications are mandated in your country, province or state. You may also want to include a paragraph about where you trained, where you have studied or under which master since, how long you have been practising, and related areas of study and experience previous to your acupuncture training.
- *A brief introduction to acupuncture and whatever other techniques are part of your practice.* In non-technical language you can explain that acupuncture, moxibustion, tui na massage, etc., correct energetic imbalances, which restores health. Again, emphasise benefits rather than features: TCM treatment gives people more energy and stamina, aids their ability to relax and sleep, reduces stress, boosts immunity, can be used in conjunction with Western medicine, etc. It is nice to know that the roots of this medicine go back 5000 years, but people have short attention spans and are mostly interested in how it is of use to them.

- *A partial list of conditions that may benefit from acupuncture.* This will help people to understand that acupuncture is not only effective for treating pain, but also many internal and external physical and spiritual–emotional conditions. You could select conditions appropriate for your geographical area and the nature of your practice from the World Health Organization's published list, or other resources.
- *Answers to the most frequently asked or most important questions.* Safety is the prime concern to people, especially the use of one-time-only disposable sterile needles. New patients may also worry about whether acupuncture is painful; you can briefly explain that most people experience nothing more uncomfortable than a small pinch, followed by a heavy or tingling sensation as the energy begins to move through the body. People also want some idea of the time and money commitment, so it is a good idea to say that when they need acute care their visits may be more frequent, but as they feel better, and the energy imbalances underlying their condition are addressed, treatments can occur less often. You may also want to mention TCM's focus on preventive health, and the benefits of occasional or seasonal tune-ups in strengthening the body's resistance to illness.

Give your brochure to each new patient; they will probably share this information with friends and family, who will see the list of things you treat that they may not know about. If they want to come and see you, they have something with your phone number on it.

At some point you will probably need to redesign your brochure to reflect changing circumstances in your practice or qualifications. For instance, if you have taken advanced studies somewhere prestigious and learned new techniques, or you've developed specialties such as treating stroke patients, or programmes for smoking cessation or infertility, you will want your patients to know that.

Distributing the brochure

You can go to community and recreation centres, libraries and health food stores, and places where you have ascertained your 'ideal' patient visits or shops, and ask for permission to display your brochure. Often these boards are cleared every 3 to 6 months and you will need to replace your material. If people you have met through your networking have premises that are connected in some way to health, they may be willing to let you put a stack on their counters. Collect feedback on your advertising by writing down where you leave brochures and noting which places display the most interest by using up your brochures more quickly. This will give you some idea about local attitudes towards natural healing.

Every time you give a public talk or lecture, whether or not the topic is general or specific, always take your brochures with you to display and to hand out. In addition, having printed material at a public lecture lends weight to your words.

Advertising in the telephone directory

If you open your practice in an area where complementary health care is not yet mainstream, you may find the Yellow Pages don't even have a category for acupuncturists! This is your opportunity to promote the credibility of the discipline, by asking the phone company to put in an acupuncture category. A listing in the Yellow Pages is often worth the expense, as people who have lost your card, can't remember your name or are looking for a new practitioner will check this first.

Establishing a website

It will come as no surprise that, in addition to asking their physician, their pharmacist or their family and friends, most people these days look for information about their symptoms or disease on the internet. Of course the reliability of the health information found on the internet is erratic, to say the least. But, for an acupuncture clinic, an informative and accessible website provides an opportunity to offer accurate, in-depth public education on TCM and the conditions it successfully treats, as well as significantly more background on the practitioner than will fit in a brochure.

The website should first and foremost introduce your training background and credentials, such as the length of your professional training, the titles you have earned and licences you have been granted, and your membership of professional colleges and associations.

Secondly, you will want to give a comprehensive explanation of the services you provide. If you have begun to focus your skills on a certain area of health, here is where you should outline your specialty. Perhaps you have had a number of women coming to see you about infertility; it is possible that you have developed a reputation as someone who can provide good results. You can then outline the treatment plan, such as explaining the use of body acupuncture, ear acupuncture or herbs and how they target the matter at hand. If you know of any articles on recent research that support the effectiveness of acupuncture in treating certain conditions, for example depression or conquering addictions, you can possibly include links to these on your site.

Patients who are happy with the results of their treatments are often willing to contribute a short testimonial. This may give you the opportunity to post a section on your site for success stories, which are informative and inspiring to potential patients.

Unless web design is among your skills, developing an effective website requires a great deal of thought and consultation with a knowledgeable and compatible designer. Look at many health-related websites to see what you like and don't like in terms of style, colour, navigability, level of detail, etc. Remember also that websites need to be maintained and links kept up to date, otherwise people will stop going there, so consider whether you have the time and energy to take on this task. If so, the website address can be included on your brochure and business card.

SETTING APPROPRIATE FEES

You cannot utilise your healing skills unless you are able to keep your office open; thus, you need to be a savvy businessperson in order to meet your financial demands. You have to earn enough money to pay rent, malpractice insurance, telephone and heating bills, regulatory body fees, continued education course fees, costs of needles and herbal supplies, and living expenses. When starting your practice, it can ease financial stress to have another part-time job to cover the basic costs of living while you build your clientele. Eventually you will have a steady flow of patients and you will probably choose to focus all your work efforts in the clinic.

On the whole, people want effective, reliable, low-risk health care. Low cost would be nice but is not often the main consideration for people making health care choices, unless their low incomes prevent them from using any kind of service that is not covered by public or private health insurance. In fact, people may not respect you or may question the quality of your service if your fee is too low.

When you move to an area, if possible find out what the current range of rates is for acupuncture treatment. You can phone colleagues in the area, ask the nearest acupuncture association, or inquire at government agencies or private insurers that fund compensation for injured workers about their fee structures for the specific service of acupuncture. If there are no other acupuncturists in the area, check the rates of physiotherapists or similar professions.

There are many factors involved in setting appropriate fees that cover your costs and earn you a decent living, while still keeping your services affordable for the local population. 'Affordable' means something different when you're working in a remote pulp mill town from what it does in a resort for wealthy retired professionals. Use all of this information to set a fair price and make your payment policy clear and easy to understand.

After a couple of years you may want to consider raising your fees. Give your patients adequate notice and do not increase fees by too much. Frequently an initial dip in patient volume occurs, but unless the fee hike has been excessive the number of patients will rebound.

RUNNING AND MAINTAINING A HEALTHY PRACTICE

A healthy practice should include a mix of new patients, long-term patients who come in regularly for seasonal tune-ups or need ongoing treatment for chronic conditions, and some in between who come for shorter courses of treatment for occasional conditions like sinus trouble or tennis elbow. Some of these patients will drop away or move; others will become long-term patients.

To keep your practice stable while continuing to update your knowledge and stay fresh, many experienced acupuncturists find that, over the long term, the ideal ratio is about 10% new patients, 40% with intermediate problems and 50% long-term patients. By long term, I mean over the course of a year or two – not that you should try to keep this exact proportion at all times.

Assessing the stability of your practice and keeping it dynamic

A tool that you may find helpful in analysing the health of your practice is, every 3 or 6 months, to make a chart as in Figure 12.1. Write the names of the months across the bottom and numbers up the left side, and plot how many patients you treat per month. After 6 to 12 months of practice, this should stabilise (Fig. 12.1a). If, however, a sudden change up or down occurs and lasts over 2 weeks (Fig. 12.1b), you should note the probable reason on the bottom of the chart. This allows you to analyse changes.

Then plot the number of *new* patients you see coming in each month. Paying attention to how many new patients are coming in will help you to assess how your practice is building. In a small area (a population less than 20000) you will probably see an increase in patient numbers up to a certain point, when you will begin to see more previous patients returning. Do not worry. This only reflects the nature of the area.

In a large urban area (more than 100 000 people), you will need to put energy towards attracting new patients. This is because people tend to be more transient owing to job changes in cities more than in rural centres.

A couple of points of clarification: do not think that any particular practice is supposed to have the numbers of patients shown on these two graphs. They are just to give an idea of the general concept and a tool with which you can analyse your practice; you can redesign it to suit yourself. The charts simply indicate trends. Also, the word 'regular' in terms of patients refers to the number of visits. If one patient comes three times in a month, it is counted as three, not one. A 'new' patient is one who is seeing you for the first time. If you're charting his third visit, for the purposes of this analytical process he is no longer considered to be a new patient, he's a 'regular'.

When the numbers of regular and new patients is roughly parallel, as in the first graph, your practice is stable. But when the number of new patients is

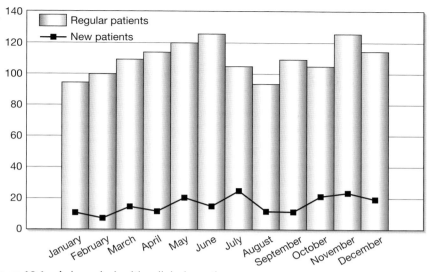

Figure 12.1a A dynamic, healthy clinical practice.

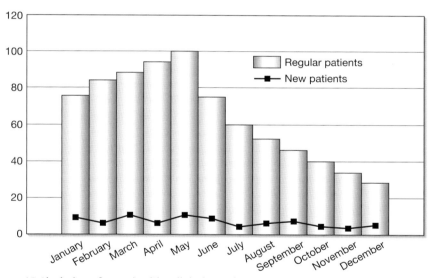

Figure 12.1b A sign of an unhealthy clinical practice.

dropping off, this is a problem. As the second graph shows, many of the long-term patients should be cured and won't necessarily be returning regularly; if there are no new ones to replace them, the practice will die.

Next, analyse the charts to see why particular results have occurred. Recognise that some factors are beyond your control: for example, summer holidays when people are away, and after Christmas when people feel financially stretched. It may also be that the local economy is doing badly and people are losing their jobs. At these times you could step up your marketing efforts by holding workshops or creating advertisements. However, if your practice is very slow for 2 or 3 months, you need to ask yourself whether there are too many practitioners in your area for the size of the population and whether your fees are too high. You may also need to take an honest look at the quality of the service you are providing (see 'Evaluating your practice', below).

If there are no obvious problems to be addressed, and your charts indicate your practice is slow and stable, then people simply must not know you. Plan some time for actions to generate more business.

Tips for generating more business

Some say that 'free' is the most powerful word in marketing and advertising for generating attention and interest. As acupuncturists, we are offering a very worthwhile service. However, giving a large number of free treatments is a sensitive issue in professional ethics; other practitioners may feel that an acupuncturist who is giving the service away is luring clients away from them. Suggested ways of using 'free' with integrity are to offer short free initial consultations, free treatments as gift certificates for community fundraising events, free educational booklets, or perhaps the first order of herbs free. Freely answering people's questions on the phone or outside the clinic also conveys a generosity of spirit.

Conduct a workshop or seminar to get your name out in public. Associations for people with cancer, heart disease, arthritis, asthma, endometriosis or infertility would probably be delighted to host you. Societies, clubs and schools, as well as intercultural associations, may also be interested. One practitioner I know moved from one side of the country to the other, where no one knew him. He visited the public library and offered to give a free lecture during allergy season on how Chinese medicine looks at allergies and how these can be treated without drugs. Many people, from seniors to young mothers, attended his lecture and subsequently booked appointments with him. This gave him a great start to his new practice.

Write articles for a local newspaper or magazines. There are often magazines that specialise in health or in particular conditions. Newsletters of support groups, such as those for men with prostate cancer, may welcome a fresh approach to the topic. Some publications want in-depth articles, whereas others may prefer a simple interview and photograph. If there is an outbreak of influenza, or some other health issue affecting your community, you could contact the local radio or TV station and offer yourself for an interview.

If you choose to place an advertisement in a newspaper or magazine, do it with a specific focus on a topic that is important for that area or at that time of year. A general ad tends to be overlooked; therefore, it is more effective to advertise on a specific subject for a short period of time. Think about what kind of people read this newspaper or magazine. A publication targeted to seniors is a good place to advertise treatments for arthritis or macular degeneration. Think of your advertising as your garden. It needs tending. Keep track of how many people phone you after reading your ad. This way you will learn how successfully you are reached by this method, and whether or not to continue.

Word of mouth is by far the most powerful form of advertising, whether the community is small or large. This is because people trust the experience of others they know. Use the network you already have by giving your business card and brochure to contacts who belong to local organisations, or patients who are about to go on a holiday with family or friends. Consider writing letters to local physicians and other health care professionals introducing yourself and indicating how you can work in a complementary way to support their patients' health.

Have educational pamphlets and books in your waiting room. These stimulate questions from your patients and their family members; remember that most people have no idea of the variety of conditions TCM can treat. They will seek your help for other health issues, and may suggest that friends or coworkers who are having health problems try acupuncture.

Focus on your practice. It is difficult to succeed if you are doing too many other things. It may be time to give up your part-time job!

Consider practising in a community where there are few complementary health practitioners. Large urban areas often have too much competition; smaller localities may need and welcome a holistic service.

Consider specialising, rather than trying to be all things to all people. It is easier to become known as an expert in infertility, chronic pain management, or adjunct care for cancer patients than as just another acupuncturist.

A strategy that often helps when business is slow is to pull out files of old clients and give them a call to find out how they are doing. Don't do this too often with the same client. You can ask patients for permission to call them in the future. They are nearly always happy to hear from you and will often book a new appointment. This is also a good way to find out whether your last prescription was effective or whether they found something else that worked better.

Analysing patient demographics and tailoring new programmes to your community's needs

If you decide your practice will benefit from focusing on a particular area of health concerns, to develop either new programmes or a long-term specialty, it is helpful to do some research to find out what your community needs most. In fact, it is informative for all new practitioners to document what sorts of conditions they have been treating over a period of time, and secondarily to have a sense of the patients' general age groups, occupations and the ratio of men and women. For the first 2 years, analyse your practice every 6 months. After 2 years, you may do this just once a year.

Make a chart listing the various conditions and the number of patients you have treated with each condition, and another showing age distribution. Finally, create a chart that shows the relative percentage of each condition in your practice.

This shows you where to devote time to studying, and it also gives you information about the nature of the community – whether there are many retired people, young families, two-career couples, etc. You will know what kind of seminars would interest this community, and what kind of articles you may want to write. Examples of perennially popular topics are allergies, colds and flu, weight loss, premenstrual syndrome, endometriosis, stress relief, chronic fatigue, headaches, diabetes and arthritis. As the 'baby boom' demographic gets older, issues such as perimenopause and menopause, prostate health and anything to do with staying young, active and sexual is likely to be of interest. So is prevention and relief of the inevitable aches and pains of the ageing body: sore knees, lower back problems and plantar fasciitis.

In order to deepen your knowledge of a particular area enough to specialise in it, you may need to study more, learn from an experienced practitioner, perhaps attend a professional development workshop, or do research interviews with a society linked to this issue.

When you are ready to open the new programme or announce your specialty, print a new brochure introducing everyone to the name of the new programme, how it works, how long it lasts, and the fee. For example, for smoking cessation you might announce 'Quit smoking with the help of acupuncture, ear acupuncture and herbs. Plan two or three visits per week for an average of three weeks for long-term heavy smokers.'

Give your new pamphlets to every patient you now have and distribute some to the locations where your new target patient population is most likely to be found.

EVALUATING THE QUALITY OF YOUR SERVICE

Whether your practice is new or established, it is beneficial to evaluate periodically how patients view your service and the quality of your care. One idea is to ask a friend or colleague who has not been your patient to assume the role of a new patient and to evaluate the experience at your office. Another possibility is to ask a neutral third party person to interview several current patients with a list of questions regarding your practice. When patients know that their opinions are given anonymously, they will feel freer to express themselves. The information revealed can be incorporated into your practice and will probably enhance patient satisfaction. Sample questions that might be included are as follows:

First contact

1. How did you find out about the office (word of mouth, telephone directory, newspaper article or advertisement, brochure, other)?
2. Were the address and telephone number clearly indicated on written material?
3. When contacting the office by telephone, were you greeted by a friendly voice and asked how you could be helped?
4. Were you placed on hold? If so, was there background music and was this agreeable to listen to?
5. Was the person knowledgeable and able to assist you?
6. Were there any words or statements made that offended you or made you think that you did not want to go to this office?
7. Were all your questions about the office answered?
8. Were the directions to the office clear and understandable, and were you told where to park?
9. Were you told what time to arrive prior to the appointment if forms were to be completed?
10. Was there a brief inquiry as to the reason for your visit?
11. Were you told how long the first visit would take and what type of payment was accepted?
12. If there was an answering machine, was the message prompt, friendly and clear?
13. How long did it take for your call to be returned (hours, days, weeks)? Did you have to call back because there was no response from the office?

Your potential patients' first verbal contact with you (or your answering machine message) can make them feel listened to – or neglected – right from the start. A bad first impression may turn patients away. Always do your best to return people's calls on the same day. Enhancing your telephone skills can

First impression of the clinic

1. Did you have any trouble finding the office (street signs clearly marked, landmarks given as directions over the phone helpful, address clearly visible from the street, sign clearly displayed)?
2. Was parking easy to find?
3. If there was a receptionist, did he or she greet you immediately and cheerfully? Did you feel welcomed?
4. Were you given instructions to fill out forms upon your arrival and shown a place to sit in order to do this?
5. Was there a place to sit in the waiting area? Was the décor pleasant and the atmosphere comfortable (furniture, colours, plants, lighting, music, reading material)?

be extremely helpful; instead of asking if they want an appointment, ask questions like 'Would you prefer a daytime or evening appointment?' or 'Would you rather come in Monday or Wednesday?'

There are two issues here. One is whether finding and getting to your clinic is as stress free as possible. If people are worrying about getting a parking ticket the whole time they are on your table, they will not be able to relax during the treatment. Detailed directions and parking information are a gift that helps patients benefit more from treatment. Secondly, the atmosphere in your waiting

The initial visit

1. Were you seen right away, or did you have to wait for a long time?
2. Did the acupuncturist introduce him or herself, greet you as Mr or Ms, and shake your hand?
3. Was the acupuncturist well dressed (clean and neat) and well groomed?
4. Was the temperature comfortable in the office?
5. Was the office clean and neat and pleasant?
6. Did the acupuncturist ask you about any fears or concerns if this was your first visit?
7. Did the acupuncturist seem organised? Were clear instructions given?
8. Were there any interruptions (telephone calls, other patients, other)?
9. Did the acupuncturist say or do anything that caused you to question his/her ability as a practitioner, or that was offensive or inappropriate?
10. Did the acupuncturist appear concerned and sympathetic to your troubles? Was there a rapport established?
11. Did the acupuncturist review your history and ask whether you had any questions?
12. Was a working diagnosis explained to you with a treatment plan?
13. If acupuncture was performed, were you comfortable with the procedure and was the experience relatively painless?
14. Did the acupuncturist explain what to expect after the treatment and as a treatment plan (likely number of treatments, frequency of treatments, duration of subsequent visits)?
15. Were you told what you could do at home to support the treatment (dietary changes, exercises or stretching, holding certain acupressure points, other)?
16. Were you given a card with the office location, phone number and next appointment time?
17. Was your financial obligation handled tactfully?
18. Did you leave feeling that you had been helped and cared for?
19. Did you feel like you used your time productively by going to this clinic? Would you go back?
20. Would you recommend this clinic to others?

area – clear signs, comfortable seating, availability of washrooms and drinking water – also contribute to patients feeling comfortable, welcome and relaxed.

An honest and detailed evaluation of the practice is not just for the new practitioner. It is something that should be done on a regular basis – at least once a year. It helps you see how many of your patients are improving and how many are still struggling. You can then ask yourself: What needs improvement? Where are my personal weaknesses and how can I work on these? Do I need to upgrade my clinical and diagnostic skills, or depth of knowledge? You may get better treatment results, and as a result more satisfied patients, simply by improving clinic management, the setup of the clinic and the direction of practice.

Each of us can develop a questionnaire appropriate to our area, culture and patients, which deepens our understanding of patients' needs as well as our own maturity of practice and ongoing commitment to our work. It is easy after many years to slide into overconfidence, laziness and an overly casual attitude that makes patients feel they've been treated in a cavalier fashion. Even after years of experience, this annual exercise of honest evaluation of self and the way we work keeps our practice fresh and motivates us to continue to learn.

Continuing education at home and abroad

13

For the TCM practitioner, homework does not end after graduation. In addition to spending time at the end of each day analysing treatments, there is a lot of reading to be done to enhance your knowledge of diagnosis and point selection.

In order to deepen your understanding, you may want to find a teacher or put together a study group to delve into the classic texts that form the foundation of TCM theory and practice. The three most important classics are: *The Yellow Emperor's Canon of Internal Medicine* (Huang Di Nei Jing), *Synopsis of Prescriptions of the Golden Chamber* (Jin Kui Yao Lue Fang Lun) and *Treatise on Febrile and Miscellaneous Diseases* (Shang Han Za Bing Lun). There are many good English translations of these. Over the years, you will find yourself returning to the 'ground' of TCM knowledge again and again.

The new practitioner is like a small tree. Once well rooted, you can absorb nutritional information from a wider circle and from different directions. After a couple of years of practice, you can attend workshops and seminars and select which new information is useful to you. These workshops can stimulate your own thinking about concepts you could adapt to your own way of practising. You can also gain information by participating in conferences, subscribing to international journals, taking part in short apprenticeships or studying in China.

APPRENTICESHIP

Apprenticeship comes in several forms. One kind is to work as part of a team with a senior practitioner. Both of you together treat a patient, and then discuss the diagnosis, treatment principles and any special techniques that may apply. You will learn a lot this way. Usually this is possible only for 2 to 6 months because it requires a lot of energy, time and agreement from patients, as well as the senior practitioner. It may be more feasible for all if this arrangement is made for a couple of days per week rather than full time, and your contribution may be to handle booking the patients.

You can learn a great deal simply by observing a senior practitioner at work. Depending on your agreement, you may ask questions discreetly during the treatment, or afterwards.

Another apprenticeship model is to practise in a second room, under the name of the senior practitioner's clinic, with your own patients and with permission to ask any questions of the senior practitioner at any time before, during or after a treatment. The senior practitioner could also teach you special techniques.

In all apprenticeships, you need to arrive at an agreement with the senior practitioner before commencing. For example, you could supply your own materials, pay rent for the room and collect all the fees from your patients; or you could use the senior practitioner's materials, and room, and pay the practitioner a percentage of each patient's fees. Your agreement should be for a specific period of time, and you should write a contract detailing matters like materials, room, how to divide patients' fees and who is responsible for booking patients.

Another way to learn from a senior practitioner is to arrange an appointment to discuss questions you may have collected from your practice. You could do this either alone or with another new practitioner. Such a meeting could involve instruction on practical techniques, case studies and diagnosis.

It is best to practise for at least 1 year before commencing an apprenticeship of any sort. That way you will already have many directed questions based on your experience. Otherwise, if you were to do it right after completing your school programme, it may seem like a continued internship and would not have as much value. You may choose to partake in different kinds of apprenticeships at different times, all depending on what works for you and your agreement with a senior practitioner.

FOCUSED STUDY

After you have been in practice for 2 or 3 years, gaining all sorts of information and firmly establishing your style, you may choose to study one or two topics intensively. In a sense, you are now choosing a specialty. Generally, your interest in a particular topic will arise from your practice. There may also be many people in your area with this condition. You may study from books, from analysing your own cases, from societies or associations that deal with this condition, from senior practitioners' experience with it, or from taking workshops. After 4 or 5 years of practising in this field, you may become one of the experts, writing articles about your chosen topic for journals and giving your own workshops.

Some people want to enrich and deepen their knowledge and skills by studying in another country. England, France, Japan, South Korea and other countries have their own tradition of acupuncture and a rich body of knowledge. If you are interested in studying in Japan, a good source of information is the *North American Journal of Oriental Medicine*, published in Vancouver, Canada. This organisation, founded for the promotion and development of Japanese approaches to Oriental medicine, puts out a publication three times a year.

Contact

NAJOM, 896 West King Edward Avenue, Vancouver, BC, V5Z 2E1, Canada; tel: 604 874-8537; website: http://members.shaw.ca/najom/Ehyoushi.htm.

How else can you find out about these special programmes? Representatives of these schools attend acupuncture and Asian medicine conferences and hold workshops to promote their programmes.

Also, your professional association will send out notices in its newsletter and have people from various schools at their national education show. The ones that are promoted through professional associations and registration bodies will have been thoroughly vetted. But be sure to check out the reputation and the roots of any other presenters or schools offering programmes. Those that have a permanent base are preferable. There are people who go around to conferences teaching some new or unusual technique, but if you then go home and start to use it, and need more information or something goes wrong, it is impossible to track them down again.

Since acupuncture originated in China, this is where it is practised most widely and for the longest time. There are many masters of acupuncture, and university and central hospital professors who take students, and many opportunities to practise with such a large population who all use this medicine. Therefore, you may well choose to go to China.

STUDYING IN CHINA

Up until the past century, in China traditional medicine was customarily learned in a family practice or apprenticeship. A vocational TCM school was opened in Shanghai in the 1930s, but closed eventually because the old pre-Mao government banned acupuncture and Chinese medicine.

Study in universities

Formal university education in Chinese medicine began to be offered in 1956. Five colleges of TCM were founded at that time, in Beijing, Shanghai, Nanjing, Chengdu and Guang Zhou. A couple of years later, a traditional medicine college was established in each of China's provinces, so there are now about 28 TCM colleges and universities.

The original schools continue to operate, and are often still academically stronger than other institutions in aspects such as student education, research and publishing. Today, they are still a good place for foreign practitioners to study; they have strong roots and each has its own specialty. You can earn a master's degree or even a doctorate at these universities.

Foreign students began to travel to China to study this exciting 'new' form of health care in the mid 1970s, after American president Richard Nixon's historic visit brought acupuncture to the attention of the Western world. Until the mid 1980s, only certain approved universities and institutes were allowed to take foreign students; now nearly all of them can do so.

The quality of TCM clinical education in China is unmatched anywhere else in the world. Because TCM is practised in Chinese hospitals as a primary care medical system, foreigners studying TCM in that country see more patients and a diversity of clinical approaches being applied to a broader variety of conditions – in a shorter period of time – than is possible in virtually any clinical setting in a Western country. In addition, learning more about Chinese culture deepens understanding of its medical tradition.

The usual application process to universities is to request an application form by mail, or to download it from the institution's website, and send it with the necessary registration fee, and a photocopy of your registration, licence or other qualifications to the overseas or foreign student office. After the application is approved, the institution will send you the letter of enrolment and other documents that you must take or send to the Chinese embassy or consulate nearest you to apply for a student visa.

The following institutions have good facilities, and skilled teaching teams including professors who speak various languages and have an understanding of the needs of foreign students. This makes the experience of study in China far less stressful.

The Beijing, Nanjing and Shanghai schools are World Health Organization Collaborative Centres on Traditional Medicine. In addition to the quality of instruction and better than average translation services they offer foreign students, they are affiliated with well-equipped hospitals.

Contact information given here does not include telephone and fax numbers, because the Chinese telecommunications system is in a constant state of upgrading and numbers change frequently. It is best to look in the English language section of the institution's website to find current numbers. Every effort has been made to include the most up-to-date internet links, but be prepared to find that email addresses also change whenever there is a new professor running the foreign student office.

The Beijing TCM University International School has an excellent reputation. Programmes for foreign students can range from a couple of months to as long as 6 years, but this school focuses on the longer programmes. Students who come from overseas often spend the first year studying the Chinese language, and in their second year join the regular classes in Chinese medicine.

Contact

Beijing TCM University International School
11 Bei San Huan East Road, Chao Yang District, Beijing, 100029, PR China;
email: isbucm@sohu.com; website: www.bjucmp.edu.cn.

The Shanghai centre is under the auspices of Shanghai TCM University's International Education School, and it has trained about 5000 TCM doctors, acupuncturists and physiotherapists from 100 countries over the past 20 years. It offers translation services in multiple languages, including English and French.

Contact

Shanghai University of Traditional Chinese Medicine, Overseas Students Office, No 530, Lingling Road, Xu Hui District, Shanghai, 200032, PR China;
website: www.shtcm.com.

Nanjing's TCM University houses the International Acupuncture Training Center where several internationally known Oriental medicine scholars and practitioners, including Giovanni Maciocia, Jeremy Ross and Julian Scott, have studied.

Contact

Nanjing University of Traditional Chinese Medicine, No 282, Han Zhong Road, Nanjing, Jiangsu Province, 210029, PR China;
website: www. iec@njutcm.edu.cn.

Two more institutions it is worth knowing about are in Chengdu and Guangzhou, because they also have a long and distinguished history of training foreign practitioners.

Chengdu University of TCM's programme ranges from a few weeks to a few months. The course format often involves working in the clinic with experienced doctors or professors each morning, and most afternoons attending lectures. This university has many doctors with a vast experience with Chinese herbs, and offers hands-on workshops in the preparation of patent herbal medicines such as pills, ointments, syrups and so on. Chengdu City is located in Sichuan province in south-west China. Sichuan province is famous for its herbs, as is evidenced in the large number of herbal names (Chuan Huang Lian, Chuan Niu Xi, Chuan Lian Zi, etc.) that include 'chuan', meaning from Sichuan. You can see lots of herbs in the local botanical garden, and there are tours available to places where you can identify herbs in their wild habitat, such as Ei Mai Mountain.

Contact

Chengdu University of Traditional Chinese Medicine, International Student Office, No 37, Shi Er Qiao Road, Chengdu, Sichuan Province, 610075, PR China; email: sqf@cdutcm.edu.cn; website: www.cdutcm.edu.cn/html/etcm.html.

Guangzhou University of TCM is a huge institution, and because of its proximity to Hong Kong has many long-standing international connections. It is considered the major TCM learning centre of the south of China, and boasts a large number of professors and doctors who are masters in their fields.

Contact

International College of Guangzhou University of Traditional Chinese Medicine, No 12, Ji-Chang Road, Guangzhou, Guandong Province, 510405, PR China; email: guoji8@gzhtcm.edu.cn; website: www.gzhtcm.edu.cn/ eindex.htm.

In addition to these five major ones, there are many cities with universities, colleges or hospital centres where foreign students can find full-service English language programmes in acupuncture and herbology. These include Tianjin, Shenyang in Liaoning Province, Harbin in Heilongjiang Province, Jinang in Shandong Province and Hangzhou in Zheijiang Province.

In choosing the most appropriate place to go, first consider large central cities versus smaller cities and towns. Foreign training centres are found only in large cities, but if you know somebody in a small town or small hospital and have a personal connection, there will be good doctors there from whom you could learn. However they may not have a residential programme, and you may need the services of an interpreter. In smaller places, you would probably have a closer relationship with the doctors, teachers and patients and you could enjoy the culture of the area.

To find out which of the many institutions will suit your needs best, it is advisable to consult with someone who knows China and the field of Chinese medicine. This could be a practitioner you know who has been to China and still has contacts, or another person who has just returned from studying in China. These people will be your most important information sources.

Nearly everywhere, you will now find amenities such as international telephone services, computers and fax machines.

Study in hospitals

For someone who wants to work more on clinical skills than enhancing theoretical knowledge, another possibility is to study in a hospital, especially a teaching hospital, rather than a university. Every big city has a TCM hospital with a full range of health care services, including traditional practitioners working in cooperation with Western-style physicians, surgeons and diagnostic tools.

The Beijing Hospital of Traditional Chinese Medicine is one of these. It originated as a clinic in a temple, and in the 1950s the hospital invited Beijing's most experienced TCM clinicians to work there. Over the years, it has built up a great reputation in Beijing; the hospital as a whole sees 4000 to 5000 outpatients, as well as 300–500 patients in the acupuncture clinic. With such a large patient population, this is a great place for an intern to study and gain clinical experience.

Generations of nationally renowned doctors have worked there and added to its knowledge base. Its cancer department, dermatological department and acupuncture department lead the country in both clinical work and research. This institution has a great deal of experience in foreign student education.

Other examples are the Tianjing Hospital of TCM, and the First Affiliated Hospital of Nanjing University of TCM. There are too many good ones to list here.

Before you go

Proposing to go to China is a big project involving much thought and preparation. You will need to give yourself enough time to gather information from people in your own country who know about China, to communicate with people in China itself, and to make economic, material and mental preparations.

You can also write a letter to the central government TCM administration bureau in Beijing for a list of programmes with well-respected doctors throughout the country.

> ### Contact
>
> Chinese National Traditional Chinese Medicine Administration Bureau, International Cooperation Department, Building No 13, Bai Jia Zhuang Dong Li, Chao Yang District, Beijing, 100026 PR China.

If you want more information about the specialties or teachers at a particular school or hospital, you can write to the TCM administration bureau of that city or region. The national administration will have those addresses, or you can even send a letter that is very generally addressed, such as 'Tianjin Traditional Chinese Medicine Bureau, Tianjin, People's Republic of China' and it will get there.

You can also write directly to each programme to find out exactly what they offer, when they start and how much they cost.

Large TCM centres are all on the internet, so you should be able to find most of the information you require by computer. The more long-standing centres will have an English website, but not all of them will, so you may need some assistance from a Mandarin speaker to navigate through these.

It is a good idea to check out three or four places unless you have a personal connection to a particular institution through someone in your own country. Compare each institution's responses to your questions, the fees, the nature of what they have to offer and your general impression.

Choosing the appropriate phase in your education for foreign study

Some graduates study in China right after their basic training, then return a couple of years later for more advanced study. Others get the most out of their trip by waiting until they have completed 1 or 2 years of practice in their own country. With some clinical experience under your belt (and, one hopes, a bit of financial stability) you then have more practical questions to ask, you know more clearly which areas you would most like to explore, and you know which areas are your weak spots where the results have not been all that good.

Do not be shy about asking the teachers to cover subject areas that reflect your particular needs and focus. You don't have to just follow the programme that is set out by the school.

Even if you have attended one of the universities, like those in Australia, that design a curriculum with some clinical work in China, it never hurts to have your own plans and priorities in mind.

It is difficult to give the cost for studying in China because the Asian markets fluctuate so much. But, as a rough guide, the tuition including translation cost for a high-standard TCM hospital, like the First Affiliated Hospital of Nanjing University of TCM, is approximately $800–1000 US/month. The prices vary depending on the size of the hospitals, the length of study and even the personal connection.

There is little opportunity to negotiate fees in a foreign student training centre. However, in hospitals and university colleges, you may find someone who is willing to help you make arrangements to teach English, or to do some computer work or other service, in exchange for some of the cost of studying Chinese medicine. You could help a professor or doctor to translate articles, assist in rewriting a Chinese medical book into English, proofread and edit a textbook, or tutor someone in order to supplement your income and to lessen the cost of your trip. Be encouraged to explore these options and do not be shy about offering your expertise in your native language.

You will enhance your ability to teach English by taking some ESL (English as a Second Language) training or certification before your trip, and take some written teaching aids with you. It would also be beneficial to familiarise yourself with TOEFL material (Test of English as a Foreign Language), an internationally recognised programme teaching vocabulary, reading comprehension, grammar and writing. Every college and university in China demands a certain TOEFL score as an entrance requirement.

Have confidence in your knowledge and skills, and also find and nourish your connections with people. If you have good interpersonal and communication skills, you can develop useful and enjoyable networks.

Recently China has passed some regulations regarding work permits for foreigners working in the country. However, if you study under the umbrella of a university or hospital, they will help you arrange ways to both study and work.

Recommended length and season of study

For most people, 3 to 6 months of studying will suffice, plus 1 month to travel and sightsee. A 1 year term may work for some people, especially if they are interested in learning a Chinese language. Spending more time will help tremendously in your future practice.

The two most enjoyable times of year are March to June and September to December. Summertime is very hot everywhere in China, and can also be humid (except Harbin, Kunming and several coastal locations). Wintertime is quite different from place to place because China is a large country north to south and from the interior to the coast. For a 6 month trip, you could go from January to early June, or from September to the pleasant springtime. The key is to avoid the hot and humid season.

There are many options in places to live, so take your time. Residential programmes are often the most expensive but convenient option. There are university student houses, university or hospital guesthouses, professors' or doctors' houses perhaps in exchange for teaching their children, and opportunities to stay with Chinese students. You could share and eat in the ordinary students' dining hall, or with a professor's or doctor's family. I suggest going to China and making your long-term living arrangements after a week or so of meeting local people, getting introduced and being exposed to the different possibilities.

The language barrier

The more Chinese language you know, the easier life in China will be, and the more benefit you will get from your study. Imagine even trying to order a meal when most restaurant menus have no English on them at all.

Learning some Chinese language, even a few basic terms like 'bu' for tonifying, will help you greatly. Many Chinese doctors have some grasp of English but it is far from fluent. Some doctors with excellent medical skills do not know any English. In any case, it is imperative that you take two dictionaries: one for general words and one for TCM terms, in both English–Chinese and Chinese–English. I recommend the following:

- *Concise English–Chinese Chinese–English Dictionary* by A. P. Cowie and A. Evison, published by The Commercial Press and Oxford University Press.
- *English–Chinese Chinese–English Dictionary of Chinese Medicine* by Nigel Wiseman, published by Hunan Science and Technology Publishing House, China. This book includes herbs.

Knowledge of the Chinese language will help you a great deal in understanding TCM concepts, and save you a fortune in interpreters! Certificates can be earned at basic, medium and high levels of the HSK (Chinese proficiency) test. Basic is just that – a vocabulary of 400 words. Different TCM courses require different levels of proficiency in language; if you are applying to do a master's or doctoral degree, you will have to have acquired at least a medium-level HSK certificate. If you have a high enough score in the HSK test, you can apply to that organisation for a scholarship for 1 to 10 months of study in China, including tuition and room and board. These scholarships are good for anything from Chinese medicine to art courses, not just language. Your nearest Chinese consulate should have information about this.

Check the requirements before you sign up for any medical courses. Language lessons are available through many universities, colleges and language institutes all over the world; the HSK tests are administered at examination centres in various countries. Information on the locations of these can be obtained at Beijing Language and Culture University; HSK Centre, email: hsk-service@blcu.edu.cn; website: www.Hsk.org.cn.

Finding a mentor and building a long-term relationship

The most valuable reward from your foreign studies goes beyond learning theory and technique. In Chinese culture, whether in arts, medicine or any other field, it is customary to establish a relationship with a 'master'. In terms of TCM, these mentors teach you while you are in China, and after you return home they will answer questions that arise for you, and perhaps help you return to pursue more advanced studies.

Generally this kind of formal declaration of a mentorship comes about after several months of studying with various masters, and establishing relationships with those whose skills and healing philosophies you admire. Some may have too many apprentices already to take on more, but others will be willing.

With Western students, the question of remuneration arises. It is appropriate to offer services in exchange for the master's teaching. Some of these include: giving English lessons to the teacher or his or her family members, helping to translate the teacher's research papers or findings, and contacting publications or international conferences on the master's behalf. Some teachers enjoy working with young people from other countries and will be happy to donate their time and expertise; others will expect help in return or even some financial offering. This is very individual. It is a good idea to reach an understanding about this to ensure neither master nor student feels advantage is being taken by the other. It never hurts to ask, politely, what the teacher would like in return for mentorship.

In addition to the personal satisfaction of deepening your knowledge, it is a boost to your professional reputation and credibility to have studied with a master.

Index

Note: page numbers in *italics* refer to figures, tables and boxes.

Referral, 152–3, 173, 178
    from physicians, 233
Registration bodies, 232
Regulatory bodies, 4, 136, 232
Remedies, 178
Ren-22, needle placement, *36*
Research interviews, 244
Responsibility in practice, 135
Romantic relationships, 145–6

Scalp acupuncture, 122
Schools, 234
Scraping tool, hygiene, 122
Self-healing mechanisms, 162
Self-injury, 92–4, 150
Seminars
    for patients, 242
    for practitioners, 249
Sensitive areas, treating, 145
Service, evaluation of quality, 244–7
Sexual ethics, 144–6
Sexual issues, 148
Sexual parts, touching, 145
Sexual relationships, 145–6
Shang Gong, 131
Shang Han Za Bing Lun *(Treatise of Febrile
        and Miscellaneous Diseases)*, 131,
        249
Shanghai school, 252, 253
Shingles, 31
Shock, 97
    arterial puncture, 36
Shu points, 193
Skin
    body defence, 89, 91
    clinical observations, 178
    needle insertion, 188–90
Skull base, needling points, 11
Small intestine, 72
SP-6
    needling angle, *27*
    uterine contractions, 106
Specialisation, 243
Specific Electromagnetic Spectrum Device,
        124
Speech impairment, 14
Spinal artery, anterior, 9
Spinal concussion, 12
Spinal contusion, 12, 15
Spinal cord, 9, 10, 13
    arachnoid cavity, 11
Spinal cord injury, 12–16
    actions, 14–15
    case studies, *12*
    prevention, 15–16
    related acupoints, *13*
    signs/symptoms, 14

Spinal nerves, 16
Spinal obstruction, 12
Spinal shock, 15
Spirit, peaceful, 110
Spiritual education, 170
Spiritual work, 144
Spleen, 77
Spleen injury, 76–8
    actions, 77–8
    case study, *76*
    prevention, 78
    related acupoints, *76*
    signs/symptoms, 77
Spleen qi deficiency, 107
Splenomegaly, 77
ST-6, electrical stimulation, 116
ST-9, needle placement, *36*
ST-19, 67
ST-36, needling angle, *26*
Standards of practice, 136
Staphylococcus, 89
Sterile conditions, 91, 92, 137
Sterilisation procedures, 90
Sternal foramen, congenital, 59–60, 61
Stomach, 69
    pathology, 70
Stomach injury, 68–71
    actions, 70
    case study, *68*
    prevention, 70–1
    related acupoints, *69*
    signs/symptoms, 70
Stomach meridian, 69
Stomach qi deficiency, 107
Storage jars, 90
Streptococcus, 89
Stress in practitioners, 226
Stroke, haemorrhagic/ischaemic, 104
Stroke patients, 16, 104
    scalp acupuncture, 122
    see also intracranial haemorrhage
Study, 249
    accommodation, 257–8
    in China, 251–9
    costs, 256–7
    different countries, 251
    focused, 250–1
    length, 257–8
    with masters, 259
    season, 257
Subarachnoid haemorrhage, 8–12
    actions, 10
    case studies, *8*
    prevention, 10–12
    related acupoints, *9, 10–11*
Subarachnoid space, 9
Subclavian arteries, 29, 30